FUNCTIONAL FITNESS FOR OLDER ADULTS

Patricia A. Brill, PhD
Functional Fitness, L.L.C.

Human Kinetics

Library of Congress Cataloging-in-Publication Data

Brill, Patricia A., 1958-
    Functional fitness for older adults / Patricia A. Brill.
        p. ; cm.
    Includes bibliographical references.
    ISBN 0-7360-4656-9 (soft cover)
    1. Exercise therapy for the aged. 2. Physical fitness for the aged.
    3. Frail elderly--Rehabilitation.
    [DNLM: 1. Exercise Therapy--methods--Aged. 2. Activities of Daily
Living--Aged. 3. Exercise--Aged. 4. Physical Fitness--Aged. WB 541
B857f 2004] I. Title.
    RC953.8.E93B75 2004
    613.7'0446--dc22   2003026202

ISBN-10: 0-7360-4656-9
ISBN-13: 978-0-7360-4656-5

Acquisitions Editor: Judy Patterson Wright; **Developmental Editor:** Elaine Mustain; **Assistant Editor:** Maggie Schwarzentraub; **Copyeditor:** Jan Feeney; **Proofreader:** Julie Marx Goodreau; **Graphic Designer:** Nancy Rasmus; **Graphic Artist:** Yvonne Griffith; **Photo Manager:** Kareema McLendon; **Cover Designer:** Jack W. Davis; **Photographer (cover):** Kelly Huff; **Photographer (interior):** Pat Brill (pp. 41, 57, 71), Dennis R. Miller (p. 107), Human Kinetics (pp. 3, 11, 31); **Art Manager:** Kelly Hendren; **Illustrator:** Katy Huggins; **Printer:** United Graphics

Printed in the United States of America   10   9   8   7

The paper in this book is certified under a sustainable forestry program.

Human Kinetics
Web site: www.HumanKinetics.com

United States: Human Kinetics
P.O. Box 5076
Champaign, IL 61825-5076
800-747-4457
e-mail: humank@hkusa.com

Canada: Human Kinetics
475 Devonshire Road, Unit 100
Windsor, ON N8Y 2L5
800-465-7301 (in Canada only)
e-mail: info@hkcanada.com

Europe: Human Kinetics
107 Bradford Road
Stanningley
Leeds LS28 6AT, United Kingdom
+44 (0)113 255 5665
e-mail: hk@hkeurope.com

Australia: Human Kinetics
57A Price Avenue
Lower Mitcham, South Australia 5062
08 8372 0999
e-mail: info@hkaustralia.com

New Zealand: Human Kinetics
P.O. Box 80
Torrens Park, South Australia 5062
0800 222 062
e-mail: info@hknewzealand.com

To D_2—For your encouragement, support, and love

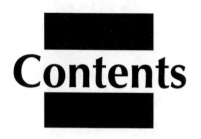

Contents

Part II   Functional Fitness Programs

Part III   Exercise Instructions and Program Guides

Program Finder

Activity program	Page numbers	Functional purposes and practical benefits	Participant characteristics	Equipment required
Lift to Function	42 108	Lower-body strength Upper-body range of motion Balance	Sedentary Uses a wheelchair for transportation Difficulty standing or walking Difficulty transferring out of chair or bed Beginning strength	Two small balls that provide resistance
Squeeze to Function	44 110	Upper-body strength Lower-body strength Range of motion and flexibility Decreases arthritis flare-ups Improves grip strength	Difficulty performing upper-body tasks such as lifting, dressing, bathing Poor balance Difficulty rising out of a chair Wants to improve leg strength to walk better Intermediate strength	Two small balls that provide resistance
Strengthen to Function	46 112	Upper-body strength Lower-body strength Range of motion and flexibility Balance	Active and semiactive Wants to improve walking and balance Wants to continue to perform daily activities Wants to improve upper- and lower-body strength Intermediate to advanced strength	Sets of two- to five-pound dumbbells Sets of one- to five-pound adjustable ankle weights Two small balls that provide resistance
Balance to Function	49 114	Improves standing and sitting balance Improves mobility and gait Improves lower-body strength, which improves balance Improves range of motion of hips and ankles Improves reaction time Decreases fear of falling Increases participation in activities	Poor sitting or standing balance Falls often or at great risk for falls Difficulty transferring out of a bed or chair Fear of falling	Large play balls Small objects Bottles or cans

Activity program	Page numbers	Functional purposes and practical benefits	Participant characteristics	Equipment required
Walk 'n' Wheel to Function	51 116	Decreases chance of dying from heart disease or cancer Improves circulation and digestion Improves resting heart rate and blood pressure Improves muscle and bone strength Improves functional performance and activities of daily living Improves strength, endurance, and balance Controls weight Improves sleep patterns Improves feelings of well-being	Wants to improve cardiovascular endurance If currently walking, or returning to walking, wants to improve stride length and step height Wants to walk greater distances	Confortable walking shoes Walking devices, as needed
Step Up to Function	58 118	Improves mobility, gait, stance, and step height Allows person to pick up feet while walking, thus less tripping Improves lower-body strength Improves circulation Improves balance, thus decreasing incidence of falls Improves transferring out of a chair Increases social participation	Poor mobility and gait Shuffles feet while walking Takes small steps while walking Trips while walking Difficulty lifting leg up into car or bathtub	Portable stair step Small ball or dumbbell
Hold It to Function	61 120	Improves lower-body strength so people can transfer and walk to the bathroom before an accident occurs Improves balance so people are less likely to fall Strengthens pelvic floor muscles so people can hold urine longer Decreases occurrences of incontinence Increases social participation	Frequent incontinence Unable to get to the bathroom in time Poor balance Difficulty walking Difficulty transferring out of a chair	None

(continued)

(continued)

Activity program	Page numbers	Functional purposes and practical benefits	Participant characteristics	Equipment required
Move to Function	62 122	Improves upper-body range of motion to help perform dressing and grooming Improves upper-body strength for eating and transferring Improves circulation in the lower legs	Bedridden Only leaves bed for meals (if then) Cannot stand on own Uses wheelchair for transportation Unable to perform many activities of daily living (e.g., dressing, bathing)	Two small balls that provide resistance
Remember to Function	65 124	Decreases wandering, agitation, physical and verbal outbursts Improves sleep patterns Improves balance (decreases falls) Allows people to perform daily activities by themselves Provides structure in daily routines Improves cognitive capacity Increases energy expenditure	Dementia or Alzheimer's disease Memory-related problems Cognitive decline Behavioral disturbances (e.g., wandering, agitation)	Large play balls Small balls that provide resistance

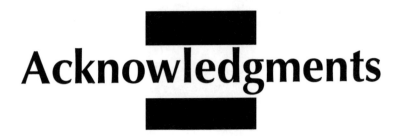

Acknowledgments

Thanks to all of the older adults I have had the privilege exercising with who showed me that with some determination, improved function is within everyone's reach. And special thanks to my friends who encouraged and supported me to be the first to write a book like this.

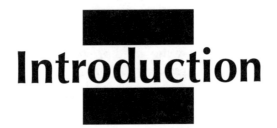

Introduction

The goal of any older adult is to remain independent and functional as long as possible. Older adults do not want to rely on others to help them dress, bathe, or perform the daily activities that they have done by themselves for many years. They want to continue to mow the lawn, travel, play with their grandchildren, and take care of themselves without help for as long as possible.

WHY USE THESE FUNCTIONAL FITNESS PROGRAMS?

Your focus as an exercise leader should be to improve the independence of your participants and help meet their functional goals. Exercise will help them meet their functional goals by improving their upper- and lower-body strength, balance, flexibility, and coordination. Falls and depression will decrease while sleep patterns will improve. Participants will be able to lead healthier, more functional lives and maintain their independence for a longer time.

Although many of you are faced with the challenge of providing exercise programs for older adults who have a multitude of chronic conditions, disabilities, and functional limitations, you may not have the training or resources to develop specific exercise programs to meet their functional needs. *Functional Fitness for Older Adults* was written to provide you and other health professionals with all of the functional fitness programs to meet the various needs of your participants within the budget of your community. These programs can be beneficial to older adults in a variety of settings such as traditional nursing homes, adult housing communities, park districts, adult day care facilities, and any other organizations or entities offering services designed to improve the health of older adults.

Because of the various levels of function of your program participants, you may need to offer different exercise programs to meet their needs. The advantage of this book is that all nine exercise programs are complete. Each program includes exercises to strengthen or stretch all of the major muscle groups used to perform daily activities. Based on scientific research, these programs have been developed to meet the various functional needs of older adults.

STUDIES ON EXERCISE-INDUCED FUNCTIONAL IMPROVEMENT IN FRAIL ELDERS

It is now clear that the beneficial effects of regular activity are observable in almost all older persons, regardless of their physical health or functional limitations. Several excellent studies have focused attention on the benefits of regular physical activity for older adults who were previously thought to be too old or too frail to participate in structured exercise programs:

• Fiatarone and colleagues (1990) conducted an eight-week, high-intensity strength training program in nine institutionalized individuals (mean age 87.9 years). Results from the study showed that strength gains increased an average of 174 percent (standard deviation was 31 percent). They conclude that high-resistance strength training can lead to significant gains in muscle strength, size, and functional mobility among frail residents of a nursing home.

• Fisher, Pendergast, and Calkins (1991) examined 18 functionally impaired nursing home residents, aged 60 to 90 years, with markedly deteriorated function. The subjects participated in a six-week strength training program. At the completion of the training program the subjects increased muscular strength by 15 percent. Many subjects increased their activity levels and decreased their dependency on others. The increase in strength was still evident four months after completion of the study. The researchers conclude that it is possible for a short-term strength training program to enhance levels of physical functioning.

• Frontera and colleagues (1988) determined the effects of strength training on muscle function and muscle mass in 12 healthy men aged 60 to 72 years. The subjects participated in a 12-week strength training program. Strength training led to muscle hypertrophy caused by an increase in type I and II fibers, which in turn led to an increase in strength.

For more such general studies on physical activity and function, see Hyatt et al. (1990), Thompson et al. (1988), Fiatarone et al. (1994), Brill (1999), Brill et al. (2000), and Huang et al. (1998).

More than 1,000 older adults residing in independent living and assisted living communities, nursing homes, and dementia care facilities have participated in the exercise programs presented in this book. All of the programs have been researched and proven effective when performed on a regular basis. Following are brief descriptions of several studies conducted with residents living in independent living and assisted living communities, nursing homes, and dementia care facilities, all of whom were involved in some of the programs in this book. Most of the research studies were conducted over an 8- to 12-week period. Subjects performed strength and balance tests before the start of the program. They then performed the same tests after the study to determine the effectiveness of the program. Objective as well as subjective results were recorded. Overall, subjects showed improvement in strength, balance, and walking speed. You will find bibliographic details in the reference list (page 127), should you wish to know the details of these studies.

• Brill, Drimmer, and colleagues (1995) selected 10 subjects (2 men and 8 women), aged 72 to 91 years (mean age 83 years), with Alzheimer's disease to study the feasibility of conducting strength and flexibility programs in elderly nursing home residents with dementia. Six different tests were administered to determine functional ability, and leg strength and functional mobility were measured by a timed chair stand test. Upper-body strength was measured by a Cybex seated chest press machine. After the training program the tests were readministered to determine whether changes in strength, flexibility, or in any other variables occurred. The study reports that a strength and flexibility training program can be successfully administered to people with Alzheimer's disease, and positive results can occur.

• Brill, Jensen, and colleagues (1998) used a randomized, controlled trial to evaluate the effect of an eight-week progressive functional fitness program on strength and functional capability in assisted living residents who used dumbbells and ankle weights. Seated chest press and leg extension strength increased 23.7 percent and 12.4 percent, respectively, in treatment group 1 (the group that exercised), compared to a decrease of 13.5 percent and 1.2 percent in treatment group 2 (the control group that did not exeircse). Performance in the timed chair stand, six-meter gait walk, and stair climb improved 24.6 percent, 11.7 percent, and 17.8 percent, respectively, in treatment group 1 compared to 20.3 percent, 13.8 percent, and 11.4 percent, respectively, in treatment group 2. A significant decrease in depression scores occurred in treatment group 1.

• Brill, Matthews, and colleagues (1998) studied 51 exercisers and 33 non-exercisers, aged 67 to 97, to determine the effect of a group-based, free weight strength training program to improve strength and functional performance among residents of two assisted living communities. A pretest and post-test design was used to measure change in strength and functional performance. Functional performance (1-time and 5-time chair stand, six-meter gait walk, balance), health perception (general health, sleep patterns, fear of falling), and medication usage were used as outcome measures. After the program, both measured functional performance and self-reported perceptions of health improved significantly among exercise participants. They also reported feeling rested when they woke up, and they rarely woke up in the middle of the night. Fear of falling decreased in the exercise participants but increased in the nonexercisers. Medication use significantly decreased in the exercisers compared to the nonexercisers.

• Brill, Probst, and colleagues (1998) evaluated the effect of an eight-week functional fitness strength training program on the functional capability in older adults. A before-and-after trial, or nonrandomized control trial, was used to conduct the program in which dumbbells and ankle weights were used. Participants were 25 volunteer residents, aged 73 to 94 years, at a multilevel retirement community. Functional performance measures (timed chair stand, six-meter gait walk, stair climb, and balance) and handgrip strength were used as the outcome measures. Overall strength, balance, and functional performance measures improved significantly. Performance in timed tests (chair stand, six-meter gait walk, stair climb, and balance) significantly improved from pre- to post-tests. This program can be used as a low-cost intervention for improving functional performance in older adults.

FEATURES IN THIS BOOK

Functional Fitness for Older Adults is organized into three parts. Part I, "Functional Fitness in Older Adults," explains how improvements in functional fitness, such as strength and balance, can help older adults perform daily activities; how to select the appropriate exercise program for your participants; exercise guidelines and safety tips; and extensive material on recruiting and motivating older adults to exercise.

Part II, "Functional Fitness Programs," includes three basic strength training programs (Lift to Function, Squeeze to Function, and Strengthen to Function), five specialized programs (Balance to Function, Step Up to Function, Hold It to Function, Move to Function, and Remember to Function) for participants with various functional needs and disabilities, and a walking and wheeling program (Walk 'n' Wheel to Function) for older adults who wish to build endurance. For optimal results, offer the specialized programs in conjunction with any of three basic strength training programs and with the walking and wheeling program.

Each strength training program incorporates exercises to strengthen major muscle groups in the upper and lower body; improve balance, flexibility, and functional performance; and provide a solid foundation for a functional fitness program for older adults. All of these programs can be conducted on an individual basis or in a group setting.

The three basic strength training programs—Lift to Function, Squeeze to Function, and Strengthen to Function—differ in terms of

- the readiness and functional capacity required of your participants,
- the type of equipment used for resistance, and
- the financial resources required.

Among the specialized programs, Step Up to Function, Balance to Function, and Hold It to Function target specific muscle groups to improve mobility, balance, and incontinence, respectively. The Move to Function program is designed for those older adults who spend most of their time in bed, possibly because of illness or muscle weakness. The Remember to Function exercise program helps decrease behavioral disturbances, such as wandering and agitation, in people who have dementia. The Walk 'n' Wheel to Function program, though structured differently from the other eight programs, provides thorough instructions on encouraging your population to get moving and keep moving so that they can continue or resume activities that have been meaningful for them in the past.

Parts I and II also include 12 true success stories taken from my experience working with older adults. These case studies not only will inspire you but will also encourage and motivate the people with whom you work, enabling them to believe that they, too, can have a better quality of life through physical activity. The more you use these programs, the more stories of your own you will collect to share with and encourage potential participants.

Part III, "Exercise Instructions and Program Guides," presents exercise illustrations, instructions, and modifications for all nine functional fitness programs. Use this section to learn how to perform each exercise correctly. Some of the illustrations of upper-body exercises feature participants using dumbbells. You can use dumbbells, balls, or no weights to perform these exercises. The illustrations for lower-body exercises feature participants using ankle weights. Again, participants also can perform these exercises without weights. To help you lead the exercise programs effectively, part III also contains visual charts summarizing each program. You may copy, enlarge, and laminate these charts. When you are conducting each program, select the appropriate chart and lay it on the floor in front of you as a handy reminder of the proper order of and technique for the exercises.

Functional Fitness for Older Adults provides you with physical activity programs that are proven to be both safe and effective for improving the functional performance levels of your participants as well as improving their health-related quality of life.

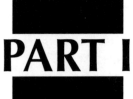

PART I

Functional Fitness in Older Adults

Most older adults want to remain independent and functional for as long as possible. As noted in the introduction, exercise provides important benefits for these older adults: cardiorespiratory functioning, maintenance of and improvement in strength and muscle mass, postural stability, and psychological functioning. Those who are already healthy can greatly increase the likelihood of remaining so, and frail and very old people can often regain these functions. By increasing bone density, coordination, balance, and muscle strength, exercise will help prevent hip fractures resulting from falls. Physical activity is also important for individuals with arthritis, Parkinson's disease, stroke, diabetes, depressive symptoms, and sleep disorders. Part I consists of three chapters that will enable you to lead older adults in exercise programs that can help them manage these conditions.

Chapter 1, "Functional Independence and Quality of Life," discusses the benefits that older adults can obtain through regular participation in a comprehensive functional fitness activity program, and how functional independence can be a primary contributor to quality of life. This chapter also presents the major muscle groups used in performing daily activities. Sharing this information with older adults can be an important part of motivating them to keep exercising. Chapter 2, "Activity Programming for Older Adults," provides guidelines to help you conduct a safe and effective activity program. Tips on recruiting and motivating older adults to remain active are included. Chapter 3, "Exercise Guidelines for People With Chronic Conditions," discusses special precautions and guidelines for older adults with specific health concerns.

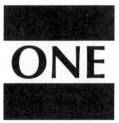

ONE

Functional Independence and Quality of Life

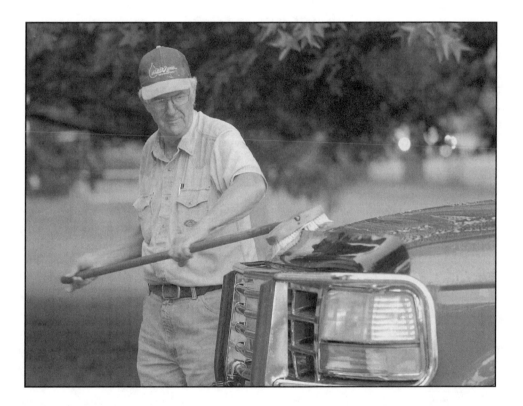

Improving functional fitness components (muscular strength, endurance, and power as well as balance, flexibility, and range of motion), whether separately or in combination, enables older adults to maintain a range of functional movement, such as climbing stairs, rising out of a chair, walking, and using a wheelchair. In turn, they are able to adopt a more active lifestyle and improve quality of life. Through effective, comprehensive functional fitness programs, older adults may be able to avoid, postpone, reduce, or even reverse declines in physical performance. Functional fitness, which determines one's ability to independently perform basic activities of daily living (ADL) such as dressing, transferring from wheelchair to bed, and bathing, should be a major factor in fitness leaders' choices of activity programs offered to older adults. This chapter discusses quality of life concerns, the benefits of becoming functionally fit, and the importance of maintaining or improving functional fitness. Primary muscle groups used in activities of daily living are identified. Lists of daily activities that use the upper and lower body are presented as well.

QUALITY OF LIFE

For many adults, growing older involves loss of strength, energy, and fitness, all of which translate to decreased quality of life. But that need not be so. The frail health and loss of function we associate with aging, such as difficulty in walking long distances, climbing stairs, or carrying groceries, are in large part due to physical inactivity. When it comes to muscle function and physical fitness, the old adage of "use it or lose it" applies. As discussed in the introduction, virtually all older adults, particularly those who are very old or frail, can improve mobility and functioning and sustain their ability to live independently with regular physical activity.

Success Story

AVOIDING THE NURSING HOME

Gloria, a resident at an assisted living facility, experienced the power of regular exercise to help her maintain the level of independence she desired. She had diabetes, chronic obstructive pulmonary disease, and peripheral vascular disease. She liked to participate in activities offered at the community; however, it was getting more difficult for her to walk to the functions because of shortness of breath, leg pain, and poor balance. She was afraid she would fall while walking down the hallways.

As time passed, Gloria became more deconditioned. She was getting to the point where she required more skilled nursing care than the assisted living community could offer. She had a choice to move to the local nursing home or to take better care of her health and remain with her friends at the assisted living facility. For months the activity director encouraged Gloria to attend the Lift to Function and Balance to Function classes. Considering her chronic conditions, the activity director knew these would be the best classes for Gloria to start out in.

At first Gloria was reluctant to participate because she was slower than the other people in the class, and she had severe cramping in her legs while performing some exercises. However, she reminded herself that she didn't want to move out of the community. At first the aides wheeled Gloria to the classes, but after only a few weeks Gloria could wheel herself. She noticed how much more arm strength she had. It was easier for her to dress and bathe herself. Eventually Gloria got to the point where she would walk to the classes using a walker. She could walk for longer periods without becoming short of breath and without pain occurring in her legs after a short distance. Gloria enjoyed participating in the classes. Because she saw such an improvement in her ability to perform the leg exercises, she performed them in her room when she got up in the morning and when she went to bed. She even began leading a little foot exercise class with the women at her lunch table.

After several months of classes, Gloria had her annual physical. Her doctor was surprised to see Gloria walk in on her own. Her hard work paid off. Gloria didn't have to move to a nursing home; she could stay in the assisted living community with her friends. Because of the tremendous change in her health and functional ability, Gloria became the community advocate for activity. Gloria strongly encourages all new residents to exercise because it can mean the difference between living there independently and moving to a nursing home.

The remarkable benefits that Gloria achieved from participating in a physical activity program may not be possible for every older adult (see "Avoiding the Nursing Home" on the previous page), but with regular, supervised physical activity, many who otherwise would lose the ability to function are able to live independently or semi-independently (perhaps in an assisted living care facility). These programs can make the difference between being bedridden and being able to do these activities:

- Play with grandchildren
- Volunteer
- Shop and go to worship services
- Travel
- Garden and do yard work
- Golf
- Go out with friends
- Cook
- Drive to doctors' appointments
- Walk to the bathroom without having to stop and rest
- Get out of a chair without help

BENEFITS OF FUNCTIONAL FITNESS

Increasing functional fitness has not only physical benefits but social and economic payoffs as well. It doesn't take much to start seeing benefits after exercising on a regular basis. Determine the needs and goals of your participants. Point out how the benefits of exercise can meet their goals.

Physical Benefits

Regular physical activity has beneficial effects on most, if not all, organ systems; consequently it prevents a range of health problems and diseases. Physical activity in older persons produces three types of health benefits:

1. It can reduce the risk of developing chronic conditions such as heart disease, diabetes, and cancer.
2. It can aid in the management of active problems such as high blood pressure, obesity, and high cholesterol.
3. It can improve a person's ability to function and remain independent in spite of health problems such as lung disease or arthritis.

Although the benefits of physical activity increase with more frequent or more intense activity, substantial benefits are evident even for those who report only moderate levels of activity. Physical activity is especially important for older men and women because they are more likely to develop chronic diseases and to have conditions such as arthritis that can affect their physical function. The potential of regular physical activity to prevent chronic diseases and sustain independence means that an active lifestyle is a key component of healthy and successful aging.

Older persons can benefit further from activities aimed at building or maintaining muscle strength and balance. A recent review of individually tailored programs for older adults demonstrates that programs designed to build muscle strength, improve balance, and promote walking significantly reduce the occurrence of falls in older persons (Gillespie, Gillespie, Robertson, et al., 2002). Experts recommend that older adults participate at least three days a week in strength training activities that improve and maintain muscular strength and endurance. Older adults also should perform physical activities that enhance and maintain flexibility. Because older adults are sensitive to the effects of physical activity, even small amounts of activity are healthier than a sedentary lifestyle.

Older adults with chronic illnesses or disabilities can gain significant health benefits with a moderate amount of physical activity, especially if it is done daily. Moderate amounts of low-impact activities such as swimming, water exercises, and stretching are recommended for those who have difficulty with their mobility.

Success Story

MOVING TO A HIGHER LEVEL

Ralph's case illustrates how exercise can enable a frail person to improve so much that he can move to a higher level of independence. Ralph was a three-year resident of a skilled care facility, having moved there because he'd fallen and broken a hip. It was difficult for him to get out of bed and move around the facility, so he just remained in bed. Both his upper and lower body became weaker. Transferring out of the bed to go to the bathroom was a chore. He was unable to bathe and dress himself as well.

Then the skilled nursing facility hired an energetic activity director, Dean, who didn't take no for an answer. Every morning he went to Ralph's room and conducted the Move to Function exercise program with him. Ralph complained, but his roommate cheered him on. He was getting stronger every day; eventually Ralph was able to get himself out of his bed and wait for Dean in his chair. One day Ralph surprised Dean by walking with his roommate to the activity room and waiting for him in one of the seats. Ralph told Dean that he was ready to progress to the Squeeze to Function class. He wanted to attend the Balance to Function class as well.

Ralph was so excited about the progress he was making, he got up early every day to dress himself and make his bed before the aides came in to wake him up. He even got so energetic that he made his roommate's bed (with him in it!). Because of Ralph's dedication to attend the classes, and Dean's persistence, he was able to do more for himself than he could do three years earlier. Ralph improved so much that he was able to move to the assisted living wing of his community. Because Ralph's roommate missed him so much, he started attending the classes as well. Now Ralph and his roommate are together again, going all about the facility on their own.

Through regular participation in the Move to Function, Squeeze to Function, and Balance to Function classes, Ralph is now able to perform the following activities of daily living:

- Bathing
- Dressing and grooming
- Walking
- Transferring out of bed
- Making the bed
- Hanging up clothes

Those who have certain disabilities can do various low-impact exercises. Some examples are wheelchair exercises and games, muscle strengthening activities to improve the ability to perform daily tasks, and strength training exercises such as light weightlifting. All of these are included in the functional fitness programs in the following chapters.

Regular physical activity has beneficial effects that are supported by the following consistent, scientific evidence:

- Lower overall mortality. Benefits are greatest among the most active persons but are also evident for people who report only moderate activity.
- Lower risk of coronary heart disease. The cardiac risk of being inactive is comparable to the risk from smoking cigarettes.
- Lower risk of colon cancer.
- Lower risk of diabetes.
- Lower risk of developing high blood pressure. Exercise also lowers blood pressure in people who have hypertension.
- Lower risk of obesity.
- Improved mood and relief of symptoms of depression.
- Improved quality of life and improved functioning.
- Improved range of motion in joint function in persons with arthritis.
- Lower risk of falls and injury.
- Lower risk of developing depression
- Improved quality of sleep

Additional possible benefits of physical activity (though research is less consistent) include the following:

- Lower risk of breast cancer
- Prevention of bone loss and fracture after the onset of menopause

Social and Economic Benefits of Physical Activity

In addition to the health and functional benefits, older persons can gain social and economic benefits through regular participation in physical activity programs. By improving mobility and functional performance, older adults are able to attend more social events in the community, go out with family members to restaurants, and visit friends and relatives without the help of others. They can remain independent in their daily activities—driving, traveling, and volunteering.

Economic benefits of physical activity are evident through lower costs for health care and medications and lower costs to live in a community (see table 1.1). That is, it costs more to live in an assisted living facility than an independent living facility, and it costs more for nursing and Alzheimer's care than for assisted living.

Community Benefits

Independent and assisted living communities, nursing homes, and Alzheimer's care facilities can benefit from offering physical activity programs as well. Programs to improve the health and functional fitness of residents can help older persons remain in their current community longer (that is, remaining in an assisted

Table 1.1 Social and Economic Benefits of Increased Functional Fitness

Functional improvement	Functional, economic, and social benefits
Improved mobility	Fewer falls, better balance, less assistance from aides
Increased range of motion	Ability to dress, groom, and bathe oneself; less work for already overburdened aides
Improved functional performance	Ability to perform activities of daily living (ADL) without assistance; less work for already overburdened aides
Greater independence	Increased self-esteem, decreased depression; increased social interaction
Increased strength and balance	Fewer falls and injuries, thus fewer costly doctor visits and hospitalization
Decreased fear of falling	Greater socialization and participation in activities
Decreased use of medication and wheelchairs; increased performance of ADL	Fewer falls, lower medication costs

living community, for example, rather than moving to a nursing home). This lowers the cost of turnover. The residents are happier, and the activity programs are a great marketing strategy. Residents who participate in activities on a regular basis will be stronger and more functional and thus more independent, requiring less time of the staff and caregivers. The caregivers can spend more time with the residents who have greater needs. In addition, healthier, more fit residents will have fewer episodes of incontinence, resulting in less work for the caregivers.

MUSCLES USED IN ACTIVITIES OF DAILY LIVING

While you are conducting a functional fitness exercise class, explain to your participants the muscles they are using and the importance of strengthening those muscles. This is an ideal time to tell them how they can improve their quality of life with these exercises.

Upper-Body Tasks

This section presents the major upper-body muscle groups stretched and strengthened throughout the activity programs. These muscle groups are instrumental in performing the following activities of daily living:

- Lifting and lowering
- Vacuuming and sweeping
- Raking leaves
- Carrying groceries
- Holding children and pets
- Bathing, using the toilet, and dressing

- Grooming
- Eating and preparing meals
- Putting away clothes
- Driving

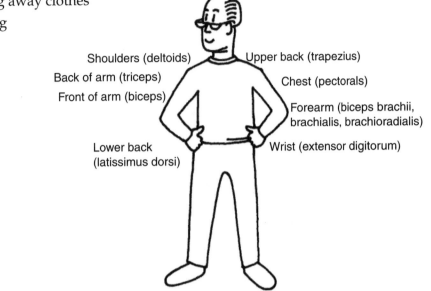

Shoulders (deltoids)
Back of arm (triceps)
Front of arm (biceps)
Upper back (trapezius)
Chest (pectorals)
Forearm (biceps brachii, brachialis, brachioradialis)
Lower back (latissimus dorsi)
Wrist (extensor digitorum)

Lower-Body Tasks

This section presents the major lower-body muscle groups stretched and strengthened throughout the activity programs. These muscle groups are instrumental in performing the following activities of daily living:

- Maintaining balance
- Walking and dancing
- Getting to the bathroom in time
- Bending
- Housekeeping
- Climbing stairs
- Doing yard work, gardening
- Transferring in and out of a chair, tub, and car

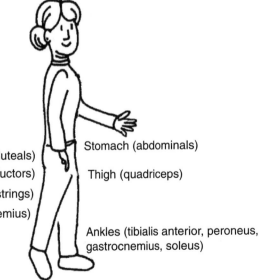

Buttocks (gluteals)
Hip (adductors, abductors)
Back thigh (hamstrings)
Calf (gastrocnemius)
Stomach (abdominals)
Thigh (quadriceps)
Ankles (tibialis anterior, peroneus, gastrocnemius, soleus)

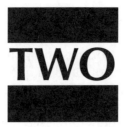

TWO

Activity Programming for Older Adults

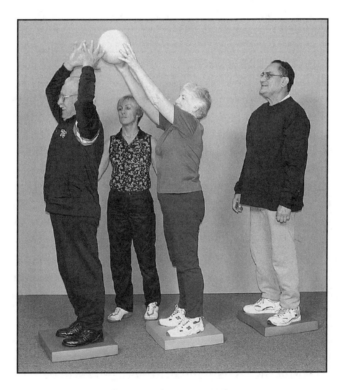

Meeting the various needs of an older adult exercise group requires attention to many details. Offering a well-rounded activity program that includes exercises to improve strength, balance, range of motion, and endurance is not enough. You must also determine the special needs of each participant before recommending programs for that person. This chapter will help you assess your participants' needs, select the appropriate programs, develop effective and safe activity programs, and motivate the older adults in your care to attend and keep attending. The result will be a healthier and happier older adult population.

ASSESSING NEEDS

Once you assess your participants' needs, you can use the program finder on page vi to select the best program. The following are steps you can take to determine the needs of your participants:

1. Older adults in any kind of exercise program should complete a brief medical history and risk factor questionnaire. A questionnaire is used to determine important information regarding potential limitations and restrictions for activity programs. Always encourage participants to consult with their health care providers if they have any questions about medical status. Use a checklist to help you gather the following essential data: medical history, physical limitations, risk factors, and medication use. If the program with which you are associated doesn't already have such a checklist, you may photocopy and use the preparticipation checklist on page 13.

2. Seek guidance from the on-site physical therapy department or the participants' health care providers.

3. Talk with participants' family members about participants' limitations.

4. Ask the participants about their medical conditions and limitations.

5. To determine the functional fitness needs of your participants, use the *Senior Fitness Test Manual* (Rikli & Jones, 2001), which provides you with simple tests to assess the functional fitness of older adults and identify people who are at risk for loss of functional mobility. Accompanying the *Senior Fitness Test Manual* is the *Senior Fitness Test Video* (Rikli & Jones, 2001). This video demonstrates seven individual fitness tests involving common activities such as getting up from a chair, walking, lifting, bending, and stretching. It also explains what equipment is needed for conducting the tests, provides safety tips, and demonstrates how to score each item. The tests have been proven safe and enjoyable for older adults, and many exercise leaders have discovered that taking the test is a motivating experience for this population. Once they see where their deficits lie, a significant number of older adults decide they want to address them, and, with the leader's help, they translate the results into realistic goals they can work toward.

6. It is also very important to conduct ongoing assessments to determine improvements and to make any necessary changes to participants' programs. Identifying and acknowledging progress is important for motivating participants to continue with their program as well as motivating others to start. Motivating your participants will be discussed at length later in the chapter.

After gathering appropriate medical history and other information, give your participants a preprogram evaluation to document baseline measures of flexibility, strength, and endurance. These measures not only will help you prescribe an appropriate activity program, but they will also encourage your participants by enabling them to measure their progress.

SELECTING APPROPRIATE PROGRAMS

As people age, they tend to lose strength and flexibility. Balance becomes worse, and falls occur. These people would benefit from strength training classes that incorporate stretching as well as low-impact endurance activities such as walking, gardening, and dancing. Many older adults may need special programs for dementia, incontinence, mobility problems, or balance.

Program Finder

Before recommending a specific activity program to a participant, you must answer some questions to determine the most appropriate program for that

Preparticipation Checklist

Name _____ Date _____

Name of physician _____ Physician's phone number _____

Medical History

___ Cardiovascular disease
___ Degenerative joint disease
___ Hypertension
___ Back pain

___ Obstructive or restrictive lung disease
___ Diabetes mellitus
___ Dizziness

Physical Limitations

___ Limited range of motion
___ Nutritional limitations

___ Mobility or balance problems
___ Risk of falls

Risk Factors

___ Family history of coronary artery disease
___ Cigarette smoking
___ Physical inactivity

___ Obesity
___ Hypertension (high blood pressure > 140/190)
___ Elevated blood lipids (cholesterol > 240 mg/dl)

Medications

___ Diuretics
___ Vasodilators
___ ACE inhibitors
___ Beta-adrenergic blockers
___ Anticoagulants
___ Digitalis
___ Lipid-lowering agents
___ Antiarrhythmic agents

___ Calcium antagonists
___ Nitrates
___ Bronchodilators
___ Antidiabetic medications
___ Levodopa
___ Nonsteroidal anti-inflamatory analgesics
___ Other

person. Ask yourself what the client's functional goals are and what types of activity programs would improve her quality of life. Second, determine whether one program will fulfill that purpose or whether two programs would be more appropriate. The program finder (page vi) uses two categories to assist you in determining the appropriate activity for each participant. Begin in the fourth column, which lists participant characteristics. When you have found a list that describes the person you're considering, look in the column immediately to the left to make sure that the list of functional purposes and practical benefits applies to this client. If these features do apply, proceed to the left to find the name and the page of the program description and the program guide that goes with it. If the functional purpose and practical benefits listed don't apply to this client, look again in the "Participant characteristics" column to see if you can find a better description of the client, and proceed from there. The last column in the Program Finder lists the equipment that each program requires.

Progression and Maintenance

Start slowly and gradually increase activity time and intensity. Most people require 4 to 6 weeks to progress from a low to moderate intensity level or level of strength. But for some, this may take 8 to 12 weeks.

Individual variability in fitness and adaptation to the exercise usually dictate the appropriate progression of an activity. Once a participant achieves a maintenance level of fitness, you may vary the regimen to enhance compliance. Most of all, emphasize enjoyment and purpose of the activity sessions.

To increase strength, your Lift to Function program participants can progress to the Squeeze to Function program, then Strengthen to Function. Bedridden participants can progress from the Move to Function to the Lift to Function program. In strength programs you can progress from using no equipment to using balls and finally to using very light weights. If very light weights are not challenging enough, you can gradually increase the weights. If a participant reaches a level where he feels he cannot progress any more, assign him as your helper to keep him active and remain with the class. If the programs you offer are not challenging enough to a participant, refer him to outside programs or a physical trainer.

ENSURING EXERCISE SAFETY AND EFFECTIVENESS

You must implement safe and effective activity programs for older adults who have multiple physical disabilities and chronic medical conditions. This section contains guidelines on conducting activity programs; emphasizing good posture, breathing, and balance; setting up your exercise space for optimal performance; ensuring the safety of your participants while they exercise; and identifying possible side effects of medications.

Basic Rules for Leading Activity Programs

Stand up or sit where you can see, as well as be seen by, all participants. You will lose participants in the back row if they cannot see you perform each exercise.

Keep a close watch on participants' technique and safety. Provide constant verbal and visual cues to describe how to perform each exercise. Remember that not every participant has good hearing or eyesight. Some people with memory loss may have difficulty following you as well. Thus, constant reminders will help them successfully perform each exercise. While participants are exercising, remind them to breathe. Sometimes they will be concentrating on doing the exercise correctly but not concentrating on breathing. Encourage participants to count along with you. This ensures that they breathe correctly, and it helps stimulate their minds. As you lead each exercise, tell your participants what muscle groups they are stretching or strengthening and how each exercise relates to their daily activities. Explaining how each exercise can help them reach their functional goals will motivate them to continue with the program. Make sure that they perform all exercises in a slow and controlled manner both for maximum effectiveness and for safety. If you are warming up or cooling down, hold each stretch 5 to 10 seconds. If you are performing strength exercises, lift for three counts, hold for one second, then lower for three counts. Offer the exercise class around the same time each day. This will help participants establish an exercise routine in their daily lives.

During standing exercises, encourage all participants at risk for falls to use chairs for support. Some might resist you and want to exercise without holding onto the back of a chair, but make sure chairs are in front of them just in case. Participants who use wheelchairs to get around but who can stand up for exercise classes should be encouraged to stand and hold the back of their wheelchair for support. Be sure the wheels are locked! (Note that some of the balance exercises presented in chapter 4 do not require a chair.)

The following guidelines are a summary of the vital procedures for leading an exercise class for older adults:

RULES FOR LEADING ACTIVITY SESSIONS

- Be sure all participants can see you throughout the class.
- Be sure you can see all participants throughout the class.
- Insist that those with potential balance problems hold onto the backs of chairs for standing exercises.
- Provide constant verbal and visual cues.
- Remind participants to breathe evenly.
- During exercises, remind participants of muscles used and their importance in daily activities.
- Do all exercises in a slow and controlled manner.
- Conduct the classes at consistent times. Establish a routine.

Posture and Breathing

When conducting an activity program for older adults, especially for chair-bound adults, incorporate both deep breathing and good posture routines to ensure maximum results. Regardless of their level of functional fitness, all participants can benefit from effective breathing and posture exercises.

Participants with respiratory disorders such as asthma, emphysema, and chronic bronchitis (all forms of chronic obstructive pulmonary disease, or COPD), as well as those with heart disease and dementia, can benefit from simple breathing exercises. Toxins are a major cause of upper respiratory infections. Deep breathing clears toxins out of the lungs, and oxygen nourishes and revitalizes body tissue. Deep breathing can also produce a relaxed state of mind. With shallow breathing, the diaphragm cannot fully expand because the rib cage collapses. Pulmonary capacity may be limited by as much as 30 percent, leading to exhaustion and irritability. Good posture facilitates proper breathing techniques by opening up the chest and allowing the lungs to expand fully. Chair- and bed-bound older adults often have shallow breathing; therefore, they especially need deep breathing and posture exercises.

Many physical problems begin with poor posture. One reason for poor posture is the dominance of one muscle group over another. An example of improper body alignment is sitting or standing slumped with the head forward and the shoulders rounded. This posture restricts the spinal nerves and, in turn, can cause numbness and weakness in the hands, arms, and fingers. If excessive neck curvature is not corrected, it can induce arthritic changes in the neck joints. When the head is directly over the shoulders, all of the muscles involved are in their proper positions. When the head slumps forward, it changes the balance of the body and puts stress on those muscles. Back spasms, neck aches, migraines, jaw pain, dizziness, and blurred vision are all indicators of how hard the body is struggling to stay upright. A rounded shoulder posture also affects the entire gastrointestinal (GI) tract, particularly the intestines. When the spine is straight, tissues hold the intestines taut in the position in which they function best. But when the spine is hunched over, the intestines can be compared to a garden hose that is constricted so that no water will come out. This inhibits the passage of the intestinal contents and can cause constipation. Correcting chair- and bed-bound older adults' posture several times a day will help them eliminate unnecessary neck and back pain, improve their breathing, and improve the functioning of their digestive systems. Body alignment plays an important role in the body's efficiency. When the body is properly aligned, the weight is balanced on all vertebrae in the spinal cord. Muscle energy is conserved, and fatigue is limited. An erect spine allows the lungs to expand fully and work to capacity, thus facilitating deep breathing.

Instruct participants to follow these guidelines to ensure good posture:

- Standing
  - Stand straight
  - Keep shoulders back
  - Keep abdomen tucked in
- Sitting
  - Sit up straight
  - Keep back against the chair
  - Keep shoulders pulled back
  - Keep feet flat on the floor

Participants must keep their feet on the floor while they are sitting and exercising. This is true even of the wheelchair-bound. If a participant's feet cannot touch the floor, place a cushion or two behind the back until the feet touch. Exercising with the feet on the floor allows participants to sit up straight. Without floor contact, exercise could place a strain on the back and neck. Shorter participants might need a small chair.

Balance

Balance involves visual, auditory, and other sensory receptors. Good balance also depends on body alignment, strength, and flexibility. Many older adults have impaired balance, which tends to reduce their sense of comfort and security. As balance becomes more of a problem to older adults, their fear of falling increases, limiting socialization and performance of daily activities. They will also reduce their risk of injury by avoiding situations that might result in a fall.

Participants with poor balance can perform the standing exercises while sitting down. Once participants get stronger and steadier on their feet, they can stand up and perform the exercises. Ask them to hold onto a chair for support if you have the slightest doubt about their stability.

Room Setup

Room setup is important for both you and the participants. Follow these general guidelines of proper room setup to minimize the chances of accidents and injuries:

- Floors in the activity room should be nonslip and free of obstructions.
- Maintain a clear path to the door for those participants who may need to leave the room if a sudden urge to void occurs.
- All balls, dumbbells, ankle weights, and other equipment should be placed under the chairs so that no one trips over them while walking through the room or while standing behind their chairs.
- Place the chairs far enough apart to give the participants enough space to perform all of the upper- and lower-body exercises without hitting other people.
- Keep class sizes small (no more than 15 residents).
- Use straight-backed chairs (if available) for good support. Chair backs should be high enough to hold onto.
- If participation results in a class size of 15 or more, offer two or more classes each day.
- Divide the participants by level of function.
- Stagger the chairs to help participants see you better, or try placing the chairs in a semicircle.
- Encourage residents in wheelchairs to use regular chairs during the session.
  - Park the wheelchairs outside the exercise room. Encouraging participants in wheelchairs to sit in regular chairs will give them a sense that they are like the other participants. Parking the wheelchairs outside will also make more room.
  - To ensure a safe transfer from the wheelchair to the regular chair, position the wheelchair next to a regular chair so that the participant can stand up and just take a step sideways in front of the regular chair and sit down. Make sure that the foot pads are in the up position and the wheels are locked before transfer.
  - If a participant has a history of falling out of a regular chair, he should remain in his wheelchair to exercise until he improves his strength and balance. When his risk for falling decreases, encourage the participant to sit in the regular chair.

- Encourage participants who remain in wheelchairs to get out of the chairs to participate in the standing exercises to help them strengthen their leg muscles and improve their balance. Make sure the wheelchairs are locked while the participants stand behind them.

It is also important to consider where each participant will sit or stand. Because routine is important, assume that participants will want to sit in the same seat every day. This makes it vital that you set up a seating pattern early in the term. Here are some things to keep in mind as you establish that pattern:

- Place participants so that everyone can see you lead each exercise. Participants will not be able to follow along and will get frustrated if they cannot see you.
- Place those with vision or hearing problems in the front of the class so that they can see and hear you and follow along with the exercises.
- If you have participants with mild memory loss or dementia, place them in the front of the class so that they can follow your lead in the exercises. At times, participants may get frustrated with those who have dementia and require more time or assistance to perform the exercises. Therefore, it might be more appropriate to have a separate class for persons with dementia.
- Place participants with weak bladders or incontinence problems closer to the door so that they will be able to leave quickly and easily.

Procedural Concerns

Here are safety precautions that are crucial to ensuring that the exercises themselves are safe:

- Always include a warm-up and plenty of stretching in each class. (See chapter 6 for details.)
- Follow the specific guidelines and exercises of each program to minimize the risk of injury and ensure a safe and effective program.
- Do not push the participants to do more repetitions or lift more weight than they can handle.
- If participants push others in wheelchairs, make sure their hands are away from the wheels.
- Develop an emergency and illness plan. Identify who should call for help.
- Participants should stop exercising if they experience any of the following symptoms:

Faintness	Numbness
Headaches	Hand tremors
Visual disturbances	Nausea
Confusion	Profuse sweating
Breathlessness	Cold, clammy skin
Nervousness	Sharp joint pain or any acute pain
Hallucinations	Irregular, rapid, or fluttery heartbeat
Unsteadiness	Fever
Chest pain	

EMERGENCY PLAN

Most residential facilities have an emergency plan in place in case a resident becomes severely ill or disoriented, falls and injures herself, or has a heart attack or stroke. To prepare for such an emergency, use the following list to form an emergency plan for your classes:

- Stop exercise immediately.
- Any participant standing should sit down.
- Have a predesignated person call the front desk and inform the staff of the incident.
- Instruct a participant to call 911.
- Clear the area around the injured participant.
- Make the participant as comfortable as possible.

Medications and Their Side Effects

The following pages contain general recommendations, practical information, and detailed medication descriptions (including potential side effects, exercise modifications, and safety precautions) reprinted by permission of the American Senior Fitness Association (1994, 2003, 2004).

Most persons with a chronic condition or disability take medications to treat their medical problems. Unfortunately, little is known about the side effects that most medications have as they relate to exercise capacity and quality of life. Some medications improve exercise performance in general, whereas some improve exercise performance when used for specific chronic diseases. However, some medications diminish exercise performance and thereby can have an adverse effect on quality of life.

Learn about the medications your participants are taking, and be able to assess how the medication may alter each person's physiology. Many older adults take several medications daily. Under these circumstances, people may forget to take their medications. Furthermore, when adherence or timing of a medication dose varies, the exercise response may be affected. As an exercise leader, you need to be aware of possible problems.

General Recommendations

Record the medications each of your participants is taking and find out the possible side effects and what you should do if they're severe. Educate yourself about how each medication may help or hinder exercise. Some medications need to be taken with meals, and other medications may be more effective if taken before exercise. For example, persons with Parkinson's disease should take their medication before exercising. The medication will help reduce the tremors and other symptoms associated with the disease.

If your facility requires you to use a medical clearance form, ask the physician whether each participant's exercise program should be restricted or adjusted because of any predictable effects of a drug regimen. A medical history form should ask participants to list all of the medications they are taking.

In some community settings, medications are administered by nursing staff. The person's care plan should take into account the potential effects of changes in medication or dosage on present activities and on recommended activity levels. As an activity director, you are responsible for obtaining all such pertinent information from medical care team members, instructing activity staff accordingly, and seeing that indicated activity programming adjustments are carried out.

If a participant's medication regimens have been altered, closely observe that participant to detect any decline in physical activity tolerance, temperature or environmental tolerance, alertness, and coordination, as well as other observable adverse reactions. If you see any such reactions, you should take immediate measures to preserve the person's health and safety.

Many older adults residing in independent and assisted living communities, nursing homes, and Alzheimer care facilities are on multiple drug regimens for two or more chronic conditions. Therefore, the likelihood for drug interaction, in addition to single-drug side effects, is much greater. Older adults often have a heightened sensitivity to a drug's intended effects and side effects. Reduced kidney function in some older adults causes drugs to clear the system more slowly than normal. In addition, physical changes brought on by age or disease make older adults three times more likely than younger persons to experience adverse side effects such as dizziness, blurred vision, and nausea (Williams 1997).

Commonly Prescribed Medications for Older Adults

You should become familiar with both nonprescription drugs and the major types of drugs commonly prescribed to older adults. Participants who want to start an activity program should discuss potential side effects with health care professionals. The more informed you are, the more able you'll be to work cooperatively with your participants and their physicians in implementing the participants' medically approved activity program, in modifying the program if necessary, and in being alert to possible signs or symptoms of medication side effects common with physical activity. You should own a comprehensive medication guidebook so that you can look up possible side effects of participants' medications.

The following descriptions of medications commonly prescribed in older populations include selected side effects that indicate practical modifications and commonsense precautions for appropriate community and long-term care activity programs.

- **ACE inhibitors** (brand name examples are Zestril and Capoten) are prescribed to treat hypertension and congestive heart failure.
  - *Side effects:* Possible side effects may include dizziness, chest pain, palpitations, muscle cramps, and joint and muscle pains. Participants on ACE inhibitors should avoid strenuous exercise as well as hot weather exercise because increased sweating or dehydration can occur, causing a rapid plunge in blood pressure.

- **Analgesics** (nonsteroidal anti-inflammatory drugs, or NSAIDs) are drugs that relieve pain. Mild analgesics, such as aspirin, may be used for conditions such as headaches and toothaches. Potent narcotic analgesics, such as morphine, are reserved for severe, persistent pain. Certain analgesics, called NSAIDs, also reduce fever and inflammation. This category of analgesics includes drugs such as aspirin, ibuprofen (brand name examples are Motrin, Advil, and Nuprin), meclofenamate (Meclomen), etodolac (Lodine), and piroxicam (Feldene). NSAIDs may be prescribed for back pain, headache, cancer pain, and gout. However they are most frequently used to treat musculoskeletal injuries and osteoarthritis.
  - *Side effects:* Side effects of NSAIDs may include gastrointestinal problems such as ulcers, kidney dysfunction, and prolonged bleeding. With NSAID use, sodium retention with weight gain and edema may also be a problem.

NSAIDs can reduce the antihypertensive effects of diuretics, beta-blockers, ACE inhibitors, and perhaps other antihypertensive drugs. Older adults on NSAIDs should be monitored for a gradually rising blood pressure and for unintended weight gain with or without edema.

- **Antiarrhythmic drugs** (brand name examples are Quinaglute, Norpace, Cordarone, Enkaid, and Mexitil) are used to control undesirable variations in heart rhythms. Generally they do so by making the muscle cells of the heart less excitable and by slowing down the conduction of electricity with the electrical system of the heart.
    - *Side effects:* Side effects may include dizziness, coordination difficulties, blurred vision, palpitations, and heightened sensitivity to sunlight. If exercising outdoors, participants taking antiarrhythmic drugs should use sunscreen, wear protective clothing, and avoid prolonged exposure to the sun.

- **Anticoagulants** (brand name examples are Coumadin and Sofarin) are commonly called blood thinners. They prevent the clotting of blood and are often used as part of the treatment process for disorders in which clot formation is dangerous, such as TIA (transient ischemic attack, or oxygen shortage to the brain), heart attack, irregular heart rhythm, pulmonary embolism, or blood clots in the limbs.
    - *Side effects:* Increased risk of bruising and hard-to-control bleeding, both internal and external.

- **Antidiabetic medications** (insulin for those with insulin-dependent diabetes and oral antiglycemic agents for people with non-insulin-dependent diabetes) are prescribed to restore the ability of the body to utilize sugar normally.
    - *Side effects:* Watch for symptoms of diabetic emergency including nervousness, shakiness, dizziness, rapid pulse, heavy sweating, excessive hunger, headache, sudden change in mood, irritability, confusion, apparent disorientation or bewilderment, reduced alertness, slurred speech, irrational or bizarre behavior, and drowsiness. Keep on hand sugar, fruit juice, candy, or other simple carbohydrates.

- **Beta-adrenergic blockers** (also known as beta-blockers) blunt the stimulating effect of the hormone epinephrine (adrenaline) on the heart, thereby reducing heart rate and contraction intensity, which decreases the oxygen requirements of the heart. Beta-blockers are used to treat hypertension, arrhythmias, angina, and in some cases migraine headaches. Many stroke patients use beta-blockers.
    - *Side effects:* General side effects of beta-blockers may include fatigue, weakness, and light-headedness. Participants on beta-blockers should avoid training programs that require standing for long periods. Because chest pain may be reduced during physical exertion, participants may tend to overexert.

- **Bronchodilators** (brand name examples are Ventolin, Alupent, and Brethine) relax bronchial smooth muscle, helping to relieve symptoms of bronchitis, asthma, emphysema, and other lung conditions.
    - *Side effects:* Side effects may include increased heart rate during exercise and heart rhythm abnormalities (irregular heartbeat, palpitations, sleeplessness, irritability, nausea, stomach pain, diarrhea, muscle twitching or spasms).

- **Calcium antagonists** (brand name examples are Cardizem, Cardene, and Procardia) are also known as calcium channel blockers. They block entry of the mineral calcium into heart muscle cells and into cells in the muscular walls of arteries. This causes the arteries to relax and keeps them from going into spasms, allowing blood to flow more easily. It also reduces the rate at which electrical impulses are conducted through the heart.
  - *Side effects:* Side effects may include edema (swelling), headache, constipation, and dizziness. Because chest pain may be reduced, participants may tend to overexert.

- **Digitalis** (brand name examples are Lanoxin and Purodigin) are often referred to by the generic names digoxin or digitoxin. They stimulate the heart to increase the force of its contractions and, in doing so, can improve the heart's pumping ability. They may be prescribed for congestive heart failure or to aid a heart muscle hindered by scar tissue after a heart attack.
  - *Side effects:* Side effects may include abnormal heart activity.

- **Diuretics** (brand name examples are Diuril and Edecrin) increase the volume of urine by promoting the excretion of salt and water from the kidneys. These medications are used to reduce edema (swelling) caused by salt retention in disorders of the heart, kidneys, liver, or lungs. Diuretics are often used in conjunction with other drugs to treat hypertension.
  - *Side effects:* Some types of diuretics may result in potassium deficiency, which can be associated with dizziness, muscle pain or cramps, muscular weakness, dehydration, and arrhythmia.

- **Levodopa** (brand name example is Larodopa) is used to treat dopamine deficiency in persons with Parkinson's disease. Levodopa enters the brain, where it is converted into dopamine, which may function as a neurotransmitter of the central nervous system.
  - *Side effects:* Older adults, particularly with a history of heart disease, are more susceptible to cardiac side effects of levodopa, such as abnormal heart rhythms. Other side effects may include muscle spasms, inability to control limb or facial muscles, nausea, loss of appetite, weakness, fainting, dizziness, and orthostatic hypotension.

- **Lipid-lowering agents** (brand name examples are Choloxin, Atromid-S, and Questran) are drugs used to lower blood cholesterol or triglyceride concentrations in persons unable to do so adequately through natural diet and exercise methods.
  - *Side effects:* Some lipid-lowering medications increase the effects of anticoagulants, placing exercise subjects at higher risk for bruising and bleeding.

- **Nitrates** (brand name examples are Nitrostat, Nitroglyn, Nitrol Ointment, and Transderm Nitro Patches) relax vascular smooth muscle, thus dilating (widening) veins and decreasing the amount of blood returned to the heart (venous return). To a lesser extent nitrates also affect arterial smooth muscle, thus decreasing the degree of resistance against which the heart must pump. In these ways, nitrates reduce the heart's workload. They are prescribed to prevent or relieve attacks of angina.
  - *Side effects:* Side effects may include flushing of the skin, headache, dizziness, and blurred vision. When nitrates are taken over a long period, orthostatic hypotension may be a problem. If one rises suddenly, more

blood remains in the extremities and less blood is made available to the brain, causing light-headedness and faintness.

- **Vasodilators** (brand name examples are Apresazide and Hydralazine) cause the smooth muscles in blood vessel walls to relax and dilate (widen), reducing resistance to blood flow and therefore making it easier for your heart to pump. Vasodilators are frequently used to treat hypertension. Coronary vasodilators may be prescribed for angina, and peripheral vasodilators may be prescribed for poor circulation in the limbs.
    - *Side effects:* Side effects may include tachycardia (an increase in heart rate above normal levels), dizziness, and orthostatic hypotension (sudden drop in blood pressure as blood supply to the brain is reduced when rising quickly from a lying or seated position).

Be aware that prescription and nonprescription drugs can cause allergic reactions. These are quite different from side effects and generally cause symptoms such as hives and rashes. Severe allergic reactions can cause breathing difficulties, shock, and even death. Report any adverse reactions to a participant's physician at once so that a decision can be made as to whether the treatment should be continued or stopped. For anyone experiencing a severe reaction, call 911 for paramedics or other appropriate emergency medical intervention.

RECRUITING PARTICIPANTS IN GROUP SETTINGS

Although educating older adults about the general benefits of exercise is an important starting point for motivating them, it is often insufficient. Even an instructor with the best exercise program may have trouble getting older adults to participate. Therefore, you must be creative in coming up with new strategies to motivate people to come to class and stick with the program. This section presents techniques and tips for motivating your participants to exercise and keep them coming back.

It is very important that you be included in the facility's admission process. When a new resident is checking in, spend a few minutes with that person and her family to introduce yourself and your programs. This is a great time to get the family involved in motivating the resident to exercise. Friends can also serve as a source of motivation. They know what tactics to use and can be very effective in motivating the resident to participate in your activity program. If you are working in a nursing home or day care center, enlist the help of the caregivers, aides, or dietary staff to recruit participants for your class. It might be more feasible to offer the class in the dining room, where people congregate before meals. Or, conduct activity programs after arts and crafts classes or sing-alongs, again when everyone is all together.

Silly as it may seem, experience has shown that older adults shy away from anything called *exercise,* and are more easily motivated to participate in what are, in fact, exercises when they are referred to as *activities* or *games.* Thus, it is important to present this not as exercise but as fun social activities and programs that can enable participants to regain or retain functions they have lost or are losing. Put it in practical terms: going out with their families, visiting home for holidays, playing with their grandchildren, resuming favorite activities they couldn't do before. Be sure their families are on board with this approach and that they understand the benefits their older relatives can get from doing these activities. Enlist their aid in talking up the *activities* (not the *exercises*). You also want to avoid the term *class.* Try *group activity* instead. Call yourself the *group leader* or *club leader* rather than the *exercise leader.* Experience shows that more older people will participate if you follow these strategies. (Note that throughout this book, we refer to *exercise.* This is acceptable among professionals, but when working with older adults avoid the term.)

Once a resident moves in, take equipment, such as balls or dumbbells, to the resident's room. Find out what activities or abilities he has either lost or is losing that he'd like to regain or maintain. Brainstorm with him on this. Point out the conditions he has that could be remedied by exercise, and explain to him how your class can help him reverse some of these declines and will help him regain or maintain his independence. Show him how you use the equipment. Address his goals, and reinforce how exercise can help meet his goals. Encourage him to join you; whether or not you get a commitment from him immediately, hang up the class schedule in his room so that he will remember the class times. Point out that he can meet new friends by attending classes.

If a resident agrees to participate, accompany the new participant to class his first day. Introduce him to the class. Give him a sense of belonging and socialization.

Visit residents who are not participating in your exercise class. Let them know you would love to have them in your class, and formally invite them to attend. Don't harass them; just let them know that they are always welcome. Promote your exercise class by having a few of your participants demonstrate the exercises at lunchtime. Occasionally ask participants to talk to other residents during lunchtime about the benefits they've experienced from the activities. Encourage participants to bring a nonexercising person to watch the class. Always announce the class over the PA system.

MOTIVATING OLDER ADULTS TO CONTINUE PARTICIPATING

The following ideas can help you keep participants from dropping out of your exercise classes. Overall strategies are presented first, and then details on using goals as motivators.

General Strategies for Motivation

The three areas to think about as you consider motivating your current and potential participants are emphasizing fun and variety in the classes, using positive reinforcement, and using any other creative strategies you can come up with.

Variety and Fun

Older adults tend to get bored by "plain" exercise. Do everything you can to bring variety and a sense of entertainment to each class.

- Play music they enjoy. Ask for their selections.
- Have a theme class (such as a luau or Halloween costume contest) every once in a while to keep your class interesting and fun.
- Share success stories frequently to encourage participants. Be upbeat and excited about these gains. You can use the case studies in this book, but also

share the successes of your own group members publicly. Congratulate them in class, and lead people in applause or even a cheer, if that seems appropriate.

- Come up with ways to make the movements a game. For example, when doing the standing leg to back exercise, you could pretend to pull your leg out of a swamp and "freeze" when tightening the buttock muscle to keep a snake from biting you until it loses interest and goes away. Or in a neck stretch, be an owl warming up its neck before going out on a nightly forage for food. Or for the chair stand, you could announce that the queen of England or president of the United States or other dignitaries are coming in and going out of a room, so you all have to keep standing up and sitting in response.

TRACKING PARTICIPATION

An essential component of an effective activity program is tracking participation.

- List all participants' names on a chart.
- Take attendance daily.
- Use stars, stickers, or other marks to denote who attended class each day.
- Have a little ceremony each day to place stickers on your chart, or have participants place check marks by their names.
- Place the participation chart where everyone can see it.
- Offer rewards for high participation:
  - Place photos up on a board.
  - Assign the privilege of being a counter or assisting in other ways.
  - Hold a lunch bunch—one day of the week when residents get to leave the community and go out to a restaurant for lunch. Most participants must be able to walk into the restaurant. Thus, a goal could be to get stronger and improve balance and mobility to be able to go to lunch.
  - Award certificates to participants.
  - Feature participants' accomplishments in a newsletter.

Positive Reinforcement

Noticing and reinforcing success in your participants will go a long way toward motivating them.

- Notice positive changes in your participants. Point out if Mary is walking faster or if John is lifting heavier weights. Let Sam know that his balance is really improving, or let LaRue know that she is now circling her ankles all the way in both directions. By pointing out little improvements, you show them you really care about them.
- Show the physicians and family members the participants' progress. Enlist these people to ask the participants about their progress and to praise their accomplishments.

- Have "Exercisers of the Month" awards. Post their names and pictures for all to see.
- Take attendance using stickers or stars. Give rewards for good attendance.
- Offer rewards for attendance and for reaching goals: certificates, T-shirts, pictures, parties, lunches, and massages.
- Use goal setting and evaluation to provide positive reinforcement. (See the section "Using Goals and Evaluation As Motivators" on the next page.)

Other Strategies

In addition to adding variety and fun to your programs, tracking participation, and providing ongoing positive reinforcement, there are other strategies you can use to help motivate participants to continue attending class on a regular basis.

Timing

One way to motivate older adults to exercise is to find the time of day that best suits their schedules and lifestyles. Some older adults find exercising first thing in the morning to be best because they don't procrastinate or get too busy and just skip it as they would tend to do later in the day. Others will want to exercise in the afternoon or evening after meals because their joints aren't as stiff as they are in the morning. It is important to find the time that participants want to exercise so that they can make it part of their daily routines.

For those older adults who have difficulty walking or are in a wheelchair but want to join your activity class, schedule the sessions for a time when you can list the help of the caregivers or aides to walk with them to the exercise room. An aide can push the wheelchair next to the participant while the participant walks.

Social Angle

Like everyone else, older adults like to have fun. Making your activity programs fun and effective will motivate participants to return time and time again. Start the class off by asking the participants what's been happening in their lives, how their grandchildren are, or what is for lunch. Allow the participants to tell something about themselves, especially if they are new, so that the class will learn about one another and will have something in common. The goals of your exercise program are to improve strength, balance, and range of motion while building camaraderie and rapport among the participants in the class. Eventually they will develop an "exercise group" and spend time together outside the activity room. Tell a joke or encourage the participants to tell a joke or a story. If someone is late, insist they tell a joke as well. The more fun they have, the more they will feel a part of the class and want to come back. Most older adults are sociable people. Make your class a positive social experience.

To increase socialization among your participants, set up a buddy system in which each participant is assigned someone for whom they are responsible to see that they get to class. Get people interacting by asking for their help. For example, assign different members to count with you, to hand out equipment or materials, or to greet new members and make them feel welcome. This not only builds social cohesion, but it also gives members a personal stake in making the group a success. If a participant misses a few classes, send her a little note to say, "We miss you."

One of the best ways that older adults can make and keep a schedule is to do it with a workout partner. Create a bulletin board, exercise chat hour, or forum to give your participants encouragement, acknowledge their successes, and celebrate their accomplishments along the way. These are also good ways to encourage other participants to join your class.

Using Goals and Evaluation As Motivators

Setting goals and monitoring and rewarding progress are the most highly motivating strategies you can use to get participants started and to keep them coming back. The best ways to motivate them to continue exercising are to help them see how exercise can be beneficial to them and to make sure that they notice or feel improvements.

Setting Useful Goals

To develop and monitor your participants' goals, you must write them down and ensure that they have certain characteristics. A good fitness goal is *specific*, *attainable*, and *measurable* (the acronym SAM). Here are some examples and guidelines for assisting your participants in setting fitness goals.

• **Specific:** A goal of lifting five pounds by the end of a six-week program is specific. Walking into church unassisted from the drop-off point at the front sidewalk to a seat in the back pew by Easter is specific. At the end of the designated time period, it will be a simple matter of determining whether the specific qualitative goal ("lifting five pounds" or "walking into church unassisted from the drop-off point at the front sidewalk to a seat in the back pew") was met within the specific time frame ("by Easter" or "in six weeks") or not.

• **Achievable:** Be sure that the goals are realistic for the participant. Don't set their sights too low, but don't set them up for failure. To set realistic goals for your participants, you will need to know their current level of function and what is possible for them to attain. If, for example, a participant's goal is to climb a flight of stairs to tuck in his grandchildren at bedtime, determine first whether he can climb stairs at all. Here are more tips for making sure goals are achievable:

  - Set a realistic date to accomplish each goal. Include the short-term goals (for example, attendance in class three times a week) that the participant must meet to achieve the final goal, and make sure that the dates and accomplishments specified for the short-term goals are realistic as well. If they aren't realistic, you may have to lengthen the overall time frame.

  - Identify factors that are now stopping the participant from reaching his goal or that could hinder him in the future, and identify strategies for overcoming them. For example, factors may include change in medications, hair or doctors' appointments, or lack of interest. If so, you could discuss with the participant's health care provider the effects of the medications and determine whether the person could take the medications earlier that day or after the exercise program. Encourage the participant to schedule the appointments later in the day or on a day when the class doesn't meet. Discuss with him the possible reasons for his dwindling interest, and then suggest solutions. Refer to the section "Using Goals to Motivate" (page 28) for guidelines on motivating older adults to exercise.

- **Measurable:** Every goal needs to include at least two measurable elements: quantity (amount of stairs to climb) and time frame (the amount of time it will take to reach the goal). Having a specific time frame also motivates participants to get started. It also helps you monitor their progress and make adjustments to the goals if necessary.

Keep the SAM acronym in mind to help you remember the basics when working with your participants to set short- and long-term goals. Start by sitting down with every new participant and helping that person articulate personal and functional goals. Help the participant think about both short-term and long-term goals. Explain to her how exercise can help her meet those goals. You may have to brainstorm with her to help her recognize the kinds of goals that are realistic for her and will improve her quality of life.

If you are working with an adult who is currently living independently, her goal may be to maintain strength and balance to be able to continue with her active lifestyle, which could involve anything from volunteering to traveling or participating in the Senior Olympics.

Older adults who are somewhat less independent may strive to improve strength to be able to climb stairs to tuck in grandchildren at bedtime, bend down to garden or perform yard work, get in and out of a bathtub without assistance from a caregiver, walk to the bathroom in time before an incontinence accident occurs, or walk without using a walker or a wheelchair. Some of your participants who have been sent to nursing homes or assisted facilities to regain motor functioning after falling and breaking a hip or having a stroke might want to get stronger so that they will be able to return to their homes to live. But none of these goals is specific or measurable, and some may not be achievable. So begin by helping all of these participants set shorter-term SAM goals that they know they need to achieve before they can reach their non-SAM goals. (If you think a particular participant will never reach that dream goal, telling her that will only discourage her. And who knows? Maybe she will reach it with your help!) The shorter-term SAM goals will vary based on each participant's level of functioning and needs. For example, for one participant, attending class three times a week for two months will help him become sturdier on his feet, thus enabling him to walk from his room to the dining area rather than being wheeled. This is a realistic shorter-term goal that would help him return to independence. As the participant meets each goal, he can maintain that goal as well as establish new goals.

Possible goals of an older adult who is bedridden or severely limited in function or mobility might be to transfer in and out of the bed or chair without assistance, walk behind a wheelchair or with a walker, and sit up straight long enough to groom herself. But every one of these at most semispecific, possibly nonachievable, and certainly nonmeasurable goals must be translated into a number of shorter-term SAM goals if the participant is to meet the general goal.

Using Goals to Motivate

List their goals privately (in their rooms) or openly (posted in the exercise room) as a reminder, and then encourage participants to support one another in achieving their goals. Tracking their attendance, recording the weights lifted and repetitions performed, or logging in the times and distances of walks all help participants see their progress in obtaining their goals. When people can see their progress in concrete terms, they are encouraged to keep going.

There may be times when participants need extra motivation. It is very common for beginning exercisers, especially those who are frail, to make fast progress at first. They might become discouraged when the improvements start to taper off. These leveling-off periods are normal, and explaining that may prevent participants from getting discouraged. Also, although they are probably doing the exercises correctly, a leveling-off period means that it is time to gradually make the activities more challenging. This might mean increasing the repetitions, weights, distance, or time.

Rewards at milestones along the way will keep your participants coming to class with their goals in view. The following are some examples of such milestones to reward: participating three times per week for six weeks, progressing to lift a predetermined weight, performing some daily activity that the person was unable to perform in the past. Each time a participant achieves a short-term goal, plan a reward and celebrate.

To work, both rewards and celebrations must be something that the participants value. A reward can be as simple as applause from the class the first time a person succeeds in walking in rather than being wheeled in, or it can be as elaborate as some of the ideas in the following list. You might need to enlist the help of participants' families to provide some of the rewards suggested here:

New walking shoes

Exercise apparel: new T-shirt, hat, shorts, walking pants, socks

Workout bag

Walking wallet or hip pack

Water bottle or holder

Walking music or workout tape

Bath time fun: scented soaps and candles, soft music, good book

Heart rate monitor or pedometer

Subscription to a walking, fitness, or health magazine

Entry into an upcoming walking event

Trip to the beach, mountains, or resort for some walking with a new view

New horn or bell for a wheelchair

Massage session

MAKING YOUR JOB EASIER

Conducting your exercise class is the easy part. The hard part is gathering up the residents, setting up the room, and getting the equipment ready for class. It can be very time consuming to gather all of your participants for exercise class, especially if many of them are in wheelchairs.

The following are tips to help you make your job easier:

- Announce the upcoming class in the hallway and in their rooms 15 to 30 minutes ahead of time and then a few minutes before the start of class.

- Recruit some of the regular exercisers to assist you. They can set up the chairs in the room, put out equipment, and knock on residents' doors to remind them of the class.

- Some participants in wheelchairs may need to be pushed to class. Assign more fit participants to bring them to class. They can be their "buddy."
- Cut out dumbbells or other pictures depicting exercise and place them next to participants' doors. Write their names and class times on the cutouts. This will remind them to exercise. The cutouts also will remind care associates to encourage them to attend class.
- Advertise in your local paper for volunteers to help with exercise classes.

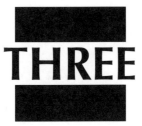

THREE

Exercise Guidelines
for People
With Chronic Conditions

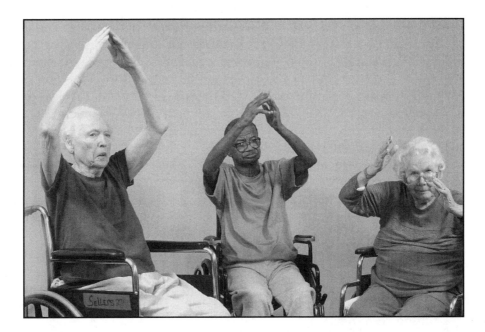

Most older adults will be able to perform any of the Fitness to Function exercises. All of the exercises are safe for older adults to perform, even if they have had a stroke or currently have heart disease, hypertension, or diabetes. However, some people with chronic medical conditions may need to modify the exercises slightly or take special precautions. All participants should inform their health care providers of their intent to exercise and the types of programs they want to do so that they can receive medical clearance to participate.

This chapter presents goals, guidelines, and suggested programs for people with the following chronic conditions:

- Arthritis
- Heart disease or hypertension
- Diabetes
- Parkinson's disease

- Stroke
- Peripheral vascular disease
- Hip fractures
- Low back pain
- Depression
- Osteoporosis

Coronary artery disease, hypertension, congestive heart failure, type 2 diabetes, osteoarthritis, osteoporosis, and cognitive disorders become more prevalent as people age. About 88 percent of people older than 65 have at least one chronic health condition, and in many cases the condition impairs function and well-being (Petrella 1999). Besides delaying the onset of many of these conditions, regular exercise may improve function and delay disability and morbidity in people who have these conditions. Given the higher incidence of these conditions with aging, even greater outcomes may be expected.

Selecting an activity program for older adults with multiple health concerns may be a challenge. It may be that they need to take two or three classes to help them reach their goals. Make a list of all of their quality of life issues and goals, and then prioritize them by the need. For example, if someone has leg weakness, a tendency to fall, and incontinence problems, he would be a good candidate for the Squeeze to Function, Balance to Function, and Hold It to Function classes. However, this person probably won't want to participate in all three classes, so select one for him to start out in. The Squeeze to Function class would be the most appropriate to start with because it works on increasing leg strength, which will help improve balance and reduce falls.

Once you select a program, call the participant's physician or send her a description and copy of the activity program her patient would like to participate in. Once the participant has his physician's approval, he can join your class. Most physicians will provide guidelines for their patients to follow.

ARTHRITIS

GOAL Increase range of motion and strength without flaring up the affected joints.

Guidelines

Tell participants that

- severe pain that does not stop after exercise suggests that there is a problem.
- if an exercise contributes to inflammation of a joint, they are performing the exercise incorrectly or with too many repetitions or too much weight.
- weight-bearing exercises should not be performed during periods of inflammation in the lower extremities.
- they should work through mild joint pain. If extreme pain occurs, they should not exercise or perform exercises that will irritate the affected joints.
- if they have rheumatoid arthritis, they should not perform the ball squeeze exercise.
- they should perform all exercises in a slow, relaxed manner.

Suggested Programs

- Lift to Function (page 42)
- Squeeze to Function (page 44)

HEART DISEASE OR HYPERTENSION

GOAL Improve functional capability and increase ability to perform activities of daily living.

Guidelines

Tell participants that

- they should avoid lifting heavy weights.
- they should not tightly squeeze the weights.
- they should alternate lifting the right and left arm.
- if anyone has a new pacemaker, she should wait eight weeks before exercising.
- they should avoid exercising in hazardous environmental conditions such as high temperatures and high humidity.
- none of them, especially those with heart disease or hypertension, should hold their breath.

Note: Some exercise experts and physicians believe that exercises involving lifting weights overhead are contraindicated in older adults with heart disease and hypertension. Discuss these exercises with your participants' physicians.

Suggested Programs

- Lift to Function (page 42)
- Squeeze to Function (page 44)
- Strengthen to Function (page 46)

DIABETES

GOAL Exercise on a regular basis. Improve cardiovascular fitness.

Guidelines

Tell participants that

- they should stop exercising if any of the following warning signs occur: faintness, headaches, visual disturbances, confusion, apathy, nervousness, hallucinations, feelings of heaviness in extremities, unsteadiness of gait, tremor of hands.
- they should not exercise on an empty stomach.
- they should eat some type of carbohydrate before exercising. Have juice on hand in case participants' sugar levels drop.
- they should avoid injecting insulin into the site of the exercising muscle.

Suggested Programs

- Lift to Function (page 42)
- Squeeze to Function (page 44)

PARKINSON'S DISEASE

GOAL Exercise on a daily basis. Improve range of motion, balance, and mobility.

Guidelines

The emphasis of the exercise program should be on improving range of motion first, then increasing strength. In addition, tell participants that they should

- use lighter weights for the strength portion of the exercise program.
- sit to perform the lower-body exercises if they have poor balance.
- wear properly fitting shoes to stabilize the heels.
- walk with a wide stance and a long stride.
- be wheeled to class to avoid fatigue if they have advanced Parkinson's disease.
- take their medications before exercising.

Suggested Programs

- Lift to Function (page 42)
- Squeeze to Function (page 44)
- Balance to Function (page 49)

STROKE

GOAL Gradually improve flexibility and range of motion in affected limb.

Guidelines

Tell participants that

- they should use lighter weights in the affected limbs.
- if they have poor balance, they should perform lower-body exercises while sitting down.
- they should lift the affected limbs as high as they can without causing extreme pain.
- they should not worry if they cannot lift the weights very high without causing extreme pain. In time, improvements will occur.

Note: Participants may not be able to regain total function, but some function will return.

Suggested Programs

- Lift to Function (page 42)
- Squeeze to Function (page 44)

PERIPHERAL VASCULAR DISEASE

GOAL Improve circulation in affected legs. Decrease pain while walking.

Guidelines

Tell participants to

- perform foot, calf, and ankle exercises two to three times per day.
- stop exercising or walking if pain occurs, then to resume exercise after two minutes.
- discuss with you and their physician whether non-weight-bearing exercises such as cycling or recumbent stepping may be more suitable for them.
- refrain from exercise when a blood clot is present.

Suggested Programs

- Lift to Function (page 42)
- Squeeze to Function (page 44)
- Balance to Function (page 49)
- Step Up to Function (page 58)

HIP FRACTURES

GOAL Increase range of motion in affected area. Gradually increase strength.

Guidelines

Tell participants

- not to use ankle weights if pain is present. When a participant is ready to use weights on the affected leg, he should start with a weight that is lighter than the weight on the strong limb.
- to lift the affected leg as high as possible without causing extreme pain.

Suggested Programs

- Lift to Function (page 42)
- Squeeze to Function (page 44)
- Strengthen to Function (page 46)
- Balance to Function (page 49)

LOW BACK PAIN

GOAL Reduce or eliminate pain in the low back area. Perform exercises with full range of motion. Increase strength in upper back, hamstrings, hip flexors, and abdominal region.

Guidelines

Make sure that participants

- lift the weights correctly.
- stand with good posture and abdominal muscles tucked in.
- avoid lifting heavy objects.

Suggested Programs

- Lift to Function (page 42)
- Squeeze to Function (page 44)

DEPRESSION

GOAL Participate in daily activities to establish a routine.

Guidelines

Suggest that participants

- exercise with partners or in a group.
- select an exercise program they will enjoy and want to participate in.
- assist you with specific tasks in the class, because this will increase their feelings of usefulness and being included in the group.

Suggested Programs

- Lift to Function (page 42)
- Squeeze to Function (page 44)
- Strengthen to Function (page 46)

OSTEOPOROSIS

GOAL Improve upper- and lower-body strength.

Guidelines

Tell participants that

- weight-bearing activities such as walking with weights and strength training are optimal. They should gradually work up to using heavier weights.
- whether standing or sitting, they should strive for good posture throughout the exercise program.

- they should inhale deeply to expand the rib cage, then slowly exhale.
- they should avoid forward flexion movements such as curl-ups.
- they should stand to perform the lower-body exercises.

Suggested Programs

- Squeeze to Function (page 44)
- Strengthen to Function (page 46)
- Step Up to Function (page 58)

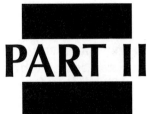

PART II

Functional Fitness Programs

Part II comprises nine fitness training programs. Chapter 4 presents activities to improve strength, range of motion, balance, and endurance, which result in increased musculoskeletal, cardiovascular, pulmonary, and functional performance levels to help older adults perform activities of daily living and improve their quality of life. All older adults, regardless of their health concerns, should be encouraged to participate in strength, balance, and endurance training. All of the programs include warm-up and cool-down exercises that address range of motion.

Chapter 5 includes Step Up to Function, Hold It to Function, Move to Function, and Remember to Function, which are specialized programs for participants with various functional needs and disabilities. Step Up to Function and Hold It to Function target specific muscle groups to improve mobility and incontinence, respectively. The Move to Function program has been designed for those older adults who spend most of their time in bed, possibly because of illness or muscle weakness. Finally, the Remember to Function exercise program helps decrease behavioral disturbances such as wandering and agitation in people who have dementia. For optimal results (that is, total fitness), you should offer the specialized exercise programs in conjunction with any of the strength training programs as well as with the Balance to Function and Walk 'n' Wheel to Function programs.

Several studies in recent years have highlighted the benefits of total fitness training for the senior population:

- Increased bone density and mass, muscular strength and endurance, flexibility, and lean muscle tissue
- Improved circulation and digestion, functional performance of activities of daily living, sleep patterns, feelings of well-being, balance, reaction time, and walking and stair climbing ability
- Decreased body fat, resting heart rate, blood pressure, chance of dying from heart disease or cancer, low-density lipid levels (bad cholesterol), and occurrence of falls and subsequent injuries

As pointed out in the introduction, research shows that all these potential physical benefits of cardiorespiratory, resistance, and flexibility exercises are real. While not as abundant, the evidence also suggests that involvement in regular exercise can provide several psychological benefits related to preserved cognitive function, alleviation of depression symptoms and behavior, and an improved perception of personal control and self-efficacy. While participation in physical activity may not always elicit increases in the traditional markers of fitness in older adults, it does improve health and functional capacity, contributing to a more healthy, independent lifestyle and greatly improving the quality of life in this population. For further information, you may want to look at two of these recent studies:

• Wood and colleagues (2001) showed that incorporating both cardiorespiratory training (such as walking) and resistance training into exercise programs for older adults may be more effective in optimizing functional fitness than using programs that involve only one component.

• King and colleagues (2000) showed that community-based programs focusing on moderate-intensity endurance and strengthening exercises or flexibility exercises can be delivered through a combination of formats that result in improvement in functional and well-being outcomes. This is one of the first studies to report significant improvements in an important quality of life outcome (in this case, bodily pain) with a regular regimen of stretching and flexibility exercises in a community-based sample of older adults.

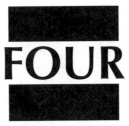

FOUR

General Functional Fitness Programs

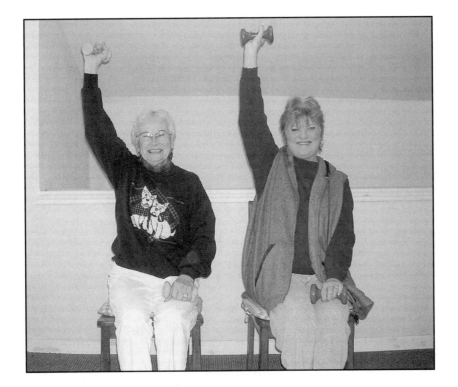

Musculoskeletal fitness is an important but undervalued component of overall health and well-being. It allows older adults to maintain functional independence. It enhances metabolic capabilities, enabling people to maintain ideal body weight. It has been shown to slow the progression of, and possibly prevent, many musculoskeletal disorders such as muscle sprains, low back pain, osteoarthritis, osteoporosis, shoulder and knee instability, and pain.

The strength training programs are listed in order of participants' level of function and in order of least to most resistance. Which programs you select will depend on the fitness level of your participants and your budget. It is recommended that all participants inform their health care providers about their intent to exercise and the types of programs they want to participate in.

Sedentary people who have difficulty standing, walking, transferring, and performing daily activities could start out in the Lift to Function program. Lift to Function uses the participant's body weight to improve upper- and lower-body strength and range of motion. Participants can improve their balance if they stand to perform the leg exercises. Those who are more mobile but have difficulty performing daily activities such as bathing or dressing should participate in the Squeeze to Function program, which uses small balls to improve upper-body strength. Leg exercises are also included, which will improve lower-body strength and balance. Those who want faster results should attend the Strengthen to Function class. This program uses dumbbells and ankle weights to improve upper- and lower-body strength, balance, and functional performance. You should offer the strength training classes at least three days per week. For optimal performance, older adults can safely participate in the strength training classes five days a week.

Included in each of the strength training activity programs are warm-up and cool-down exercises. These exercises are vital for maintaining and improving range of motion and functional performance in older adults. Improved flexibility enables adults to better dress and bathe themselves, reach for grocery items on top shelves, and drive cars.

LIFT TO FUNCTION

Lift to Function is a seated exercise program that uses the participant's body weight to help strengthen major muscle groups in the upper and lower body, as well as improve range of motion.

Success Story

SLIMMER AND HAPPIER

Mary Jean, aged 75 and a very sociable resident of the assisted living facility, always had a weight problem. It wasn't until she started participating in the activity classes that she began to lose weight. Remarkably, as the weight came off, her medication requirements changed. She was able to stop taking some medications and reduce the dosages of other medications. She now has more energy for social activities and has more money to spend on fancy dresses and hats.

Features of Lift to Function

The Lift to Function program includes 3 arm exercises to improve upper-body strength and 10 leg exercises to improve lower-body strength. Participants can improve balance by standing to perform the leg exercises.

The Lift to Function program

- uses body weight for resistance,
- is a seated exercise program,
- provides sitting modifications to the standing exercises, and
- is a short exercise program (less than 30 minutes long).

The main **focus** of Lift to Function is to improve lower-body strength. This will help participants stand up for longer periods, walk greater distances, and transfer out of chairs. This program is great for beginners and those in wheelchairs who have difficulty standing, walking, transferring, and performing daily activities.

A **participant** who will benefit from this program

- may be sedentary,
- may use a wheelchair for transportation,
- could have difficulty standing or walking, or
- has difficulty transferring out of a chair or bed.

The following are **practical benefits** of Lift to Function:

- Improved lower-body strength increases standing time, walking distance, and ease of transferring out of a chair.
- Improved upper-body range of motion increases ability to do daily activities such as bathing, dressing, grooming, and toileting.
- Improved balance increases participants' ability to stand to perform the leg exercises.

The improvements in lower-body strength, upper-body range of motion, and balance also will increase participants' ability to take part in and enjoy social activities.

Here are the **guidelines** to follow as you lead this program:

- Perform 3 to 5 repetitions of each warm-up and cool-down.
- Perform 10 repetitions of each upper- and lower-body exercise.
- Participants with poor balance should sit to perform the lower-body exercises.

The **equipment** required for the Lift to Function program is two small balls that provide resistance. These balls will be used in the ball squeeze exercise.

Success Story

A WALK TO REMEMBER

Leonard was a very active resident, always dancing with the ladies at social functions. One day Leonard suffered a stroke, which limited him to walking only short distances. Previously his granddaughter had asked Leonard to walk her down the aisle at her wedding. He thought he would never be able to do this and became depressed. After many discussions with the activity director, he decided that participating in the Strengthen to Function and Balance to Function classes might help him improve his mobility and reach his goals. After months of hard work, Leonard was able to walk his granddaughter down the aisle and dance with her at her wedding. Now Leonard has many ladies lining up to dance with him once again.

Lift to Function Program Elements

Here are the exercises for the Lift to Function program. The program guide for Lift to Function is on page 108, and the page numbers where the description of each exercise can be found are noted after each exercise in the following lists:

Warm-Up

Shoulder circles, page 72

Neck stretch, page 72

Arm stretch, page 73

Back squeeze, page 75

Wrist circles and extensions, page 76

Ball squeeze, page 80

Sitting Exercises

Arm press and pull, page 79

Chair lift, page 79

Reverse curl, page 87

Leg extension, page 89

Leg squeeze, page 89

Circle and point, page 91

Chair stand, page 98

Lower-Body Exercises

Heel and toe, page 91

Knee raise, page 93

Leg to side and cross, page 94

Leg to back, page 95

Leg curl, page 95

Squats, page 97

Cool-Down

Shoulder circles, page 72

Arm push, page 74

Back squeeze, page 75

Hugs, page 76

Wrist circles and extensions, page 76

Deep breathing, page 78

Maintaining Lift to Function Gains

To help your participants maintain or even improve the functional abilities they gained through the Lift to Function program, encourage them to attend the Squeeze to Function or the Strengthen to Function class. If participants do not want to progress, make sure they still attend the Lift to Function class on a regular basis.

SQUEEZE TO FUNCTION

Squeeze to Function incorporates 10 ball exercises to improve upper-body strength as well as 7 leg exercises to improve lower-body strength and balance. Compared to the Lift to Function program, Squeeze to Function includes more arm exercises and the use of balls for resistance. This helps improve participants' upper-body strength at a greater rate.

Features of Squeeze to Function

The Squeeze to Function exercise program uses two small balls for resistance to improve upper-body strength.

Other features are that the program

- includes standing leg exercises to improve lower-body strength and balance,
- provides sitting modifications to the standing exercises,

Success Story

STRONG ENOUGH TO HELP

Mr. Miller used to walk around the cafeteria helping others open up their milk cartons and juice bottles. He would also use this time to socialize. But after a while he started having difficulty with this task, so he stopped. Because he couldn't help others anymore, he stopped socializing and became depressed. One day the activity director stopped to talk with Mr. Miller. After determining what was happening, the director encouraged Mr. Miller to attend the Squeeze to Function class. He told Mr. Miller that by participating on a regular basis, he would see an improvement in his grip strength, which would help him perform fine motor movements such as opening milk cartons and jars. Shortly after going to the Squeeze to Function class, Mr. Miller was back socializing around the cafeteria, opening jars, and recruiting residents to the class.

- progresses easily into the Strengthen to Function program, and
- is a short exercise program (less than 30 minutes long).

The main **focus** of Squeeze to Function is to improve upper-body strength, which is important for daily tasks such as lifting and carrying groceries, bathing and dressing, transferring out of a chair, and doing yard work. The Squeeze to Function program also helps participants improve lower-body strength and balance.

The **participant** who will benefit from this program

- has difficulty performing upper-body tasks such as lifting, dressing, and bathing;
- has poor balance;
- has difficulty rising out of a chair; and
- wants to improve leg strength to walk better.

The following are **practical benefits** of Squeeze to Function:

- It is a total body program.
- Ball exercises improve upper-body strength for daily activities such as
    - lifting and lowering,
    - bathing,
    - dressing, and
    - carrying heavy items.
- Ball exercises help decrease arthritis flare-ups.
- Ball exercises increase grip strength, which facilitates fine motor movements such as opening milk cartons or jars and buttoning clothes.
- Leg exercises build lower-body strength to improve
    - gait,
    - mobility, and
    - transferring.
- Improved range of motion increases ability to do activities of daily living.

Here are the **guidelines** to follow as you lead this program:

- Perform 3 to 5 repetitions of each warm-up and cool-down.
- Perform 10 repetitions of each upper- and lower-body exercise.
- Squeeze the ball before performing each exercise.

The **equipment** required for this program is two small balls that provide resistance.

Squeeze to Function Program Elements

Here are the exercises for the Squeeze to Function program. The program guide for Squeeze to Function is on page 110, and the page numbers where the description of each exercise can be found are noted after each exercise named in the following lists:

Warm-Up

Shoulder circles, page 72

Neck stretch, page 72

Arm stretch, page 73

Arm push, page 74

Wrist circles and extensions, page 76

Chair stand, page 98

Upper-Body Exercises

Ball squeeze, page 80

Roll and press, page 80

Top and bottom press, page 81

Shoulder squeeze, page 81

Lateral raise, page 83

One-arm row, page 84

Biceps curl, page 85

Wiper, page 85

Reverse curl, page 87

Abdominal twist, page 87

Lower-Body Exercises

Leg squeeze, page 89

Leg extension, page 89

Circle and point, page 91

Heel and toe, page 91

Leg to side and cross, page 94

Leg curl, page 95

Squats, page 97

Cool-Down

Shoulder circles, page 72

Arm push, page 74

Back squeeze, page 75

Hugs, page 76

Wrist circles and extensions, page 76

Deep breathing, page 78

Maintaining Squeeze to Function Gains

Those who participate in Squeeze to Function can easily progress to the Strengthen to Function program because the exercises are similar. The only difference is that Strengthen to Function uses dumbbells and ankle weights for resistance, whereas Squeeze to Function uses balls.

STRENGTHEN TO FUNCTION

The Strengthen to Function program uses dumbbells and ankle weights. It includes nine exercises to improve upper-body strength and nine exercises to

Success Story

A THANKSGIVING SURPRISE

While recruiting residents to participate in the Strengthen to Function program, the activity director met a woman named LaRue, aged 87. LaRue told the activity director, "I would like to walk again. My doctor said I should just accept being in this wheelchair but I can't. I want to walk by Thanksgiving, and I believe that your strength training program will help me to achieve my goal." LaRue attended the Strengthen to Function program five days a week from July until November. Her motivation and dedication to achieving her goals paid off. During the four-month period, LaRue progressed from using a wheelchair to using a walker and then to using just a cane. On Thanksgiving day, LaRue walked into her family's house carrying a pumpkin pie. LaRue never told her family she was participating in a strength training program on a regular basis to help her walk. So when they saw her walk into the room, unassisted and carrying a pie, they screamed, LaRue screamed, and she dropped the pie. The family was so excited, everyone cried.

improve lower-body strength. It is also a progressive program. For example, participants will start performing 8 repetitions of each exercise the first week. In the second week they will perform 10 repetitions, then 12 repetitions the third week. In the fourth week they will drop back to 8 repetitions but increase the weight of the dumbbells and ankle weights.

Features of Strengthen to Function

The features of Strengthen to Function are that it

- is a total body program,
- uses dumbbells and ankle weights for resistance,
- progresses in repetitions and amount of weight,
- produces faster results than the Squeeze to Function program,
- provides sitting modifications to the standing exercises, and
- has 30- to 40-minute classes.

The main **focus** of Strengthen to Function is to improve upper- and lower-body strength, balance, flexibility, and coordination in older adults who participate in this program on a regular basis. This program also has the potential to reverse functional loss, thus improving activities of daily living, maximizing functional skills, decreasing the need for assistance, and enabling participants to maintain independence.

The **participant** who will benefit from this program

- is active,
- wants to improve walking and balance,
- wants to continue to perform yard work or gardening tasks, and
- wants to continue sports participation such as golf or fishing.

The following are **practical benefits** of Strengthen to Function:

- Improved upper-body strength helps older adults perform daily activities such as lifting and lowering, bathing, dressing, and carrying heavy items.
- Enhanced lower-body strength improves gait, mobility, and transferring.
- Improved balance helps prevent falls.
- Improved range of motion increases ability to do activities of daily living.
- Improved functional performance enables older adults to live independently.
- Participation in social activities increases.

Here are the **guidelines** to follow as you lead this program:

- Tell participants not to squeeze the dumbbells.
- For optimal benefits, encourage participants to work out at least three days per week. Also encourage them to increase the weight as they progress; lifting the same weight week after week won't stress the muscles or bones, so strength gains will not occur.
- Perform all of the strength exercises in a slow and controlled manner.
- Lift the weights for three counts, hold, then lower for three counts.

The following is the required **equipment** for this program:

- Dumbbells (sets of two, three, four, and five pounds)
- Ankle weights (adjustable one to five pounds per ankle)
- Two small balls that provide resistance

Strengthen to Function Program Elements

Here are the exercises for the Strengthen to Function program. The program guide for Strengthen to Function is on page 112, and the page numbers where the description of each exercise can be found are noted after each exercise named in the following lists:

Warm-Up

Shoulder circles, page 72

Neck stretch, page 72

Arm stretch, page 73

Back squeeze, page 75

Wrist circles and extensions, page 76

Ball squeeze, page 80

Upper-Body Exercises

Shoulder press, page 82

Front raise, page 82

Lateral raise, page 83

Upright row, page 84

One-arm row, page 84

Biceps curl, page 85

Triceps extension, page 86

Reverse curl, page 87

Abdominal twist, page 87

Maintaining Strengthen to Function Gains

To help your participants maintain or even improve the functional abilities they gained through the Strengthen to Function program, encourage them to progress further by increasing the weight of the dumbbells or ankle weights. If your participants do not want to increase weights, make sure they still attend the Strengthen to Function class on a regular basis.

BALANCE TO FUNCTION

Poor balance, limited mobility, and falls are the main reasons older adults become more dependent and obtain the services of home health care, adult day care centers, assisted living communities, and nursing homes. The combination of lower-body strength (including ankle strength and flexibility and good mobility) and good balance is critical in decreasing the risk of falls and maintaining functional independence.

Success Story

SHE COULD HAVE DANCED ALL NIGHT

Genie and Joe liked to dance together at all of the events at their assisted living community. They would be the first up to dance and the last to leave. Periodically, Genie would lose her balance while walking to the social hall or while dancing. This concerned Genie and her family and led to Genie's significantly cutting back on her repertoire of dance steps. Through the encouragement of her family and the activity director, Genie started to attend the Balance to Function class on a regular basis. After just a few weeks, Genie's balance improved so much, she and Joe were back on the dance floor twirling around and dipping every now and then. Other residents were so impressed at Genie's improvement that they signed up for the Balance to Function class as well. Now hardly anyone sits down at the social events.

Features of Balance to Function

The Balance to Function program has eight individual and six group activities to help older adults improve vertigo and balance. Exercises strengthen the leg and back muscles, thus improving balance and mobility. In addition, participants perform exercises to increase range of motion in hips and ankles.

Other features are that the program

- is developed specifically for people who have poor standing or sitting balance,
- decreases the risk for falls and subsequent injuries,
- is a short exercise program (less than 30 minutes long).

The main **focus** of Balance to Function is to improve steadiness in standing, sitting, walking, and transferring.

The **participant** who will benefit from this program

- has poor sitting or standing balance,
- falls often or is at great risk for falls,
- has difficulty transferring out of a bed or chair, or
- has a fear of falling.

The following are **practical benefits** of Balance to Function:

- Improved standing and sitting balance decreases the number of falls.
- Increased lower-body strength improves
    - balance,
    - mobility, and
    - gait.
- Improved range of motion increases ability to do activities of daily living.
- Improved reaction time.
- Decreased fear of falling.
- Increased participation in activities.

Here are the **guidelines** to follow as you lead this program:

- Offer the Balance to Function class at least twice per week.
- Place participants in a group setting far enough apart so that they have their own space.
- Always have support, such as a chair or a wall, next to the participants while they perform the standing balance exercises.
- Encourage slow movement at first.
- Perform three to five repetitions of each warm-up and cool-down.

The following is a list of **equipment** required for this program:

- Large ball for each participant
- Six small objects (e.g., plastic ice cubes, dice, pens)
- Bottle or can for each participant

Balance to Function Program Elements

Here are the exercises for the Balance to Function program. The program guide for Balance to Function is on page 114, and the page numbers where the description of each exercise can be found are noted after each exercise named in the following lists:

Warm-Up

Shoulder circles, page 72

Neck stretch, page 72

Arm stretch, page 73

Arm push, page 74

Back squeeze, page 75

Wrist circles and extensions, page 76

Individual Exercises

3-Stance, page 100

Foot stand, page 101

Step right and left, page 101

Ball pass, page 101

Tandem walk, page 102

Foot alphabet, page 102

Group Exercises Standing in a Line

Overhead ball pass, page 103

Ball pass between legs, page 103

Alternate head and legs, page 103

Ball pass to side, page 103

Group Exercises Sitting in a Circle

Pass the tray, page 104

Object pick-up, page 104

Side pick-up, page 104

Cool-Down

Shoulder circles, page 72

Arm push, page 74

Back squeeze, page 75

Hugs, page 76

Wrist circles and extensions, page 76

Deep breathing, page 78

Maintaining Balance to Function Gains

Encourage residents who are at risk of falling to participate in the Balance to Function class as well as the Lift to Function, Squeeze to Function, or Strengthen to Function classes. Offer the Balance to Function class two times per week or incorporate the balance exercises into other exercise classes.

WALK 'N' WHEEL TO FUNCTION

The 1996 Surgeon General's report, "Physical Activity and Health," recommends "a minimum of 30 minutes of physical activity of moderate intensity on most, if not all, days of the week." The benefits are greatly reduced risk of heart disease, diabetes, cancer, stroke, and other maladies. Walkers have also been shown to continue to be active in their later years and to live longer. Walking is inexpensive, requires little equipment, can be done almost anywhere, and is good for young and old alike.

You can use four facets to help your participants set up a new habit for a lifetime. First, help them set clear and realistic goals. Second, keep them on a schedule so that the habit sticks. Third, monitor their progress and reward them for success. And fourth, keep it interesting. You may have to constantly motivate your participants to keep them in the program to reach their goals.

Success Story

GONE FISHING

Ed, a new resident of the assisted living facility, approached the activity director to request that she help him walk again. Ed had been using a wheelchair for a couple of years. Diabetes and poor balance were the reasons he used wheelchair. His motivation to walk was based on his passion for fishing. If Ed couldn't walk to the boat, he would not be able to go fishing. So a determined Ed worked hard every day to strengthen his legs and improve his balance. We notified the staff at a local department store of Ed's goal to walk again. The store donated a gift certificate for Ed to use once he could walk into their store to shop for fishing supplies. Well, the day came. The activity director took Ed to the store to pick out his fishing pole. Unbeknownst to Ed, the store had a red carpet laid out from the parking lot into the store for Ed to walk across. Ed was so surprised and happy that he could finally fish again. Later that day, Ed caught a 12-inch catfish.

Note that older adults in wheelchairs can also improve their cardiovascular endurance and upper-body strength by participating in walking programs. For these people the "walking" is modified to "wheeling."

As you learned in chapter 2, the essentials of a good fitness goal are making it realistic, measurable, and attainable. A walking goal should be challenging but realistic. Don't set their sights too low, but don't set them up for failure, either. To set realistic and measurable goals for your participants, you will have to know their current level of function and what is possible for them to attain. If a participant's goal is weight loss, do not set a goal of losing more than 1 to 2 pounds a week or 5 to 10 pounds a month, and plan for plateaus along the way. For increasing speed and distance, participants should plan to increase no more than 15 percent per week to prevent injury and allow muscles to repair and strengthen. Their goals should be stated in a way that can be measured. What is the distance they would like to walk at one time, or how many miles a week? How many pounds or inches would they like to lose? By what date? Set dates by which they can attain their short-term goal and intermediate goals along the way.

How often to walk or wheel: Repetition is the key to building a habit. Making a schedule and tracking it are essential in a walking program. Older adults should walk or wheel a minimum of three times per week (that is, every other day) for 20 to 30 minutes. For those older adults who have difficulty walking short distances, they should walk several times a day, each time increasing the distance. Eventually these participants will be able to join the Walk 'n' Wheel to Function program.

When to walk or wheel: You must find the time of day that best suits participants' schedules and lifestyles so that they can make walking or wheeling part of their daily routines. For those older adults who have difficulty walking or are in a wheelchair but want to start walking, enlist the help of caregivers or aides to walk with them to each meal. An aide can push the wheelchair next to the participant while the participant walks. An older adult should set a goal to walk a little farther to each meal. Some older adults who do not find walking or wheeling particularly enjoyable prefer to get their aerobic exercise in first thing in the morning. That way they "get it over with" before they get too busy and just skip it as they would tend to do later in the day. Still others walk in the afternoon or evening after meals. One of the best ways to make and keep a schedule is to do it with a walking partner; companionship acts as a motivator to get out the door. Creating a walking 'n' wheeling club, bulletin board, or walking chat hour can give your participants encouragement and a way to celebrate along the way. It is also a good means of recruiting other participants to walk or wheel.

Recording participants' walks or wheels is the best way to maintain motivation. To help your participants track their walks and wheels and progress, print out monthly walking calendars or weekly walking logs for participants to use as daily walking or wheeling journals or for memories of each walk.

Positive rewards at milestones along the way will keep your participants' walking or wheeling habits fresh and their goals in view. The following are some examples of such milestones to reward:

- Weight loss. Every five pounds toward a weight loss goal earns a reward.
- Distance. If the goal is to reach a certain distance, divide that goal into quarters. Each time a participant achieves a quarter-goal, celebrate.
- Time. If the goal is to increase walking time, divide the goal time into quarters and celebrate each time a participant has achieved another quarter toward the goal. For example, if the participant wants to be able to walk for 20 minutes, celebrate his ability to walk 5 minutes, 10 minutes, 15 minutes, and then 20 minutes.
- Schedule. Each week that a participant sticks to her walking schedule, plan a reward and celebrate (refer to pages 25 and 55 for ideas).

Features of Walk 'n' Wheel to Function

Participants in the Walk 'n' Wheel to Function program can perform individually or as a group. People who use any type of assisted device can participate in this program, and they should be encouraged to do so.

The main **focus** of Walk 'n' Wheel to Function is to improve participants' cardiorespiratory fitness levels. Participants who walk on a regular basis will be able to strengthen muscles and bones; improve balance; and improve their function in performing daily tasks such as bathing, dressing, and grooming.

The **participant** who will benefit from this program

- wants to improve stride length and step height,
- wants to walk greater distances, or
- wants to improve cardiovascular endurance.

The following are **practical benefits** of Walk 'n' Wheel to Function:

- It decreases the chance of dying from heart disease or cancer.
- It improves circulation and digestion.
- It improves resting heart rate and blood pressure.
- It improves muscle and bone strength.
- It improves blood lipid levels.
- It improves functional performance and performance of ADL.

- It improves
  - strength,
  - endurance, and
  - balance.
- It controls weight.
- It improves sleep patterns.
- It improves feelings of well-being.

Here are the **guidelines** to follow as you lead this program:

- Instruct participants to stand up straight with the chin up while walking.
- Instruct participants to swing arms at a 90-degree angle.
- Encourage participants to maintain a good stride while walking.
- Remind participants to breathe while walking.
- Add time and distance to goals.
- Encourage participants to walk 20 to 30 minutes a day.

The **equipment** required for this program is a pair of comfortable walking shoes. Multiple medical and physical problems can make walking difficult; various walking devices are available to make walking safer, easier, and less painful. Walkers, canes, and wheelchairs probably will be required for some participants.

- **Walkers.** A walker is usually necessary for severe balance problems and can be useful if bearing weight on one leg is painful. If a stroke has left a participant with a weak hand, you or the participant can order a platform (arm rest on side of walker) or a hemi walker (a smaller walker with four legs to use with the strong hand). If a person has difficulty walking long distances, strategically place a chair or bench so that she can sit and rest before continuing her walk.

- **Canes.** Compared to regular, single-point canes, quad canes (canes with four feet) provide more stability and support for an unsteady person. Single-point canes are helpful for those who have slight balance difficulties or need mild support for a painful leg. Both types of canes have handles that come in a variety of shapes and forms. For a person with arthritis, there are canes with special handles that mold to a person's grip.

- **Wheelchairs.** People in wheelchairs should especially be encouraged to walk. If someone is afraid to use a walker, he can walk behind his wheelchair for support. Once he gets tired, he can sit down in his chair or in a nearby chair. Always have someone walk beside a person walking with a wheelchair.

Safety Tips

Because the walking activities will not always be done in the context of a class, it is especially important to emphasize to participants the following safety tips:

- Wear comfortable, supportive walking shoes.
- Walk on even, hard surfaces.
- Do not walk alone, especially at night.

- Do not walk during extreme heat, humidity, or cold.
- Warm up and cool down before and after each walk.
- Drink plenty of water before, during, and after each walk.

Walk 'n' Wheel to Function Program Elements

Here are the warm-up and cool-down exercises for the Walk 'n' Wheel to Function program. The program guide for Walk 'n' Wheel to Function is on page 116, and the page numbers where the description of each exercise can be found are noted after each exercise named in the following lists:

Shoulder circles, page 72

Neck stretch, page 72

Back squeeze, page 75

Quadriceps stretch, page 77

Calf stretch, page 77

Abdominal twist, page 87

Side bends, page 88

Circle and point, page 91

Heel and toe, page 91

Maintaining Walk 'n' Wheel to Function Gains

The only way to maintain function in this program is to keep walking! Following are strategies that can help you motivate your participants to do just that:

- Establish a walking club in your community.
- Use a chart to record the distance and time participants walked.
- Place the chart where everyone can see it.
- Set distance goals, and chart participants' progress to reach these goals. Create an accumulated mileage program that records the number of miles walked in a facility and gives participants credit for each mile. Draw a map and mark off the distance that participants cover each day.
- Provide incentives such as certificates, ribbons, medals, or lunch out of the facility for reaching certain points along their travels.
- Feature a walker of the month.
- Pair up people based on their walking speed.
- Provide participants with personal walking charts to monitor their progress.
- Set up walking stations throughout the route. Have posters displaying the exercise you want your participants to perform. For example, participants could perform wall push-ups at one station.

For more walking games and activities, read *Walking Games and Activities: 40 New Ways to Make Fitness Fun,* by June Decker and Monica Mize (Human Kinetics 2002).

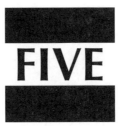

FIVE

Fitness Programs for People With Functional Disabilities

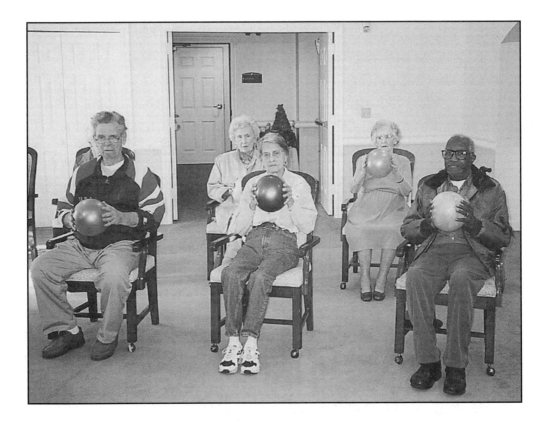

This chapter presents four specialized exercise programs for older adults who have balance and mobility problems, incontinence, limited range of motion, arthritis, and dementia. Some of these programs could be offered in conjunction with one of the five basic functional fitness programs presented in chapter 4.

STEP UP TO FUNCTION

Loss of muscle mass and leg strength makes it more difficult for a person to walk long distances or walk at a normal pace. Those with tight hip muscles or weak leg muscles may have difficulty lifting up their legs, so they shuffle their feet. This causes them to be at greater risk for falling and suffering subsequent injuries. These people also will have difficulty getting in and out of cars or bathtubs.

Features of Step Up to Function

The Step Up to Function program includes a series of steps up and down on a step and six lower-body standing exercises to improve leg strength, balance, and mobility. The program also includes five foot exercises for circulation.

The main **focus** of Step Up to Function is to strengthen major muscle groups in the lower body to improve gait speed and height and stair climbing ability.

The **participant** who will benefit from this program

- has poor mobility and gait,
- shuffles the feet while walking,
- takes small steps while walking,
- trips while walking, and
- has difficulty lifting legs up into a car or bathtub.

The following are **practical benefits** of Step Up to Function:

- It improves mobility, gait, stance, and step height.
- It enables participants to pick up their feet while walking, thus avoiding tripping.
- It improves lower-body strength.
- It improves circulation.
- It improves balance and decreases falls.
- It improves ability to transfer out of a chair.
- It increases social participation.

Success Story

CRUISING ON VACATION

Grace, a resident of an independent living facility in Columbia, South Carolina, wanted to go on an Alaskan cruise. She knew that to keep up with her family members she would have to increase her strength and stamina. Grace religiously attended the Step Up to Function program for four months before the cruise. At last the day came for her to go on the cruise. When she returned, she reported to the other participants in her class that she outdanced everyone on the cruise. She also climbed the stairs to daily activities instead of taking the elevator. Passengers on the cruise as well as her family were surprised to see how much energy she had for an 86-year-old woman. Grace said her greatest accomplishment was climbing up an iceberg to get her picture taken.

Here are the **guidelines** to follow as you lead this program:

- Instruct participants to maintain good posture while stepping.
- Instruct participants to lean forward slightly while stepping up.
- Encourage participants to relax the shoulders.
- Instruct participants to avoid locking the knees.
- Participants should wear shoes that have firm traction and provide support to the arches and ankles.
- Step height for beginners should start at the lowest level (approximately four inches).
- Foot placement is very important. Feet should always point straight ahead, and weight should be distributed along the whole foot.
- When demonstrating the steps, place the entire foot on the center of the platform when stepping up. Step ball to heel.
- When stepping off the platform, place the sole of the foot on the floor. Step ball to heel.
- Participants should hold onto the back of chairs while stepping.
- If participants start hitting the side of the step, have them sit and step or sit and rest.
- Participants may sit to perform the stepping series. Gradually progress the participants to stand and step.
- One repetition is equal to this: Step up on right foot, then left foot; then step down on right foot, then left foot.
- Follow the weekly step guide. For example, in week 1 perform five steps with the right foot and five with the left foot. In week 2 perform six steps with the right and six with the left foot, and so on.
- Once participants complete the 12-week step program they can maintain stepping 16 steps per repetition.

The **equipment** required for this program is a stair step and a small ball or dumbbell.

Step Up to Function Program Elements

Here are the exercises for the Step Up to Function program. The program guide for Step Up to Function is on page 118, and the page numbers where the description of each exercise can be found are noted after each exercise named in the following lists:

Warm-Up

Shoulder circles, page 72

Neck stretch, page 72

Arm stretch, page 73

Arm push, page 74

Back squeeze, page 75

Wrist circles and extensions, page 76

Foot Exercises

Circle and point, page 105

Toe and heel tap, page 105

Foot roll, page 105

Scrunch and wiggle, page 106

Sole press, page 106

Step-Up Routine 1

Perform the appropriate step-up routine from the 12-Week Stepping Program, step-up routine 1 (below), starting with the right foot.

Lower-Body Exercises

Perform the following exercises starting with the right foot. Then repeat them all, starting with the left foot.

Heel and toe, page 91

Knee raise, page 93

Leg to side and cross, page 94

Leg to back, page 95

Leg curl, page 95

Squats, page 97

Step-Up Routine 2

Perform the appropriate step-up routine from the 12-Week Stepping Program, step-up routine 2 (below), starting with the left foot.

Cool-Down

Shoulder circles, page 72

Arm push, page 74

Back squeeze, page 75

Hugs, page 76

Wrist circles and extensions, page 76

Deep breathing, page 78

Maintaining Step Up to Function Gains

To maintain the gains acquired through participation in the Step Up to Function program, participants can progress to the Strengthen to Function class. The Strengthen to Function program will help them maintain their lower-body strength while they improve their upper-body strength.

12-WEEK STEPPING PROGRAM

Step-up routine 1:   Step up, starting with the right foot.

Week	1	2	3	4	5	6	7	8	9	10	11	12
Number of steps	5	6	7	8	9	10	11	12	13	14	15	16

Step up: Right foot up, left foot up.

Step down: Right foot down, left foot down.

Step-up routine 2: Repeat stepping, starting with the left foot.

Week	1	2	3	4	5	6	7	8	9	10	11	12
Number of Steps	5	6	7	8	9	10	11	12	13	14	15	16

Step up: Left foot up, right foot up.

Step down: Left foot down, right foot down.

HOLD IT TO FUNCTION

People suffering from incontinence typically have weak lower-body muscles and poor balance; therefore, they are unable to get to the bathroom in time once an urge to void occurs. The Hold It to Function class can help your participants deal with their incontinence.

Success Story

REGAINING CONTROL

Mildred shied away from social activities in the nursing home because she had urinary incontinence. She didn't like to be far from a bathroom. On repeated occasions the activity director tried to persuade Mildred to attend the activity class specifically designed for people with incontinence. Reluctantly Mildred agreed to try a class, and then she continued to attend class on a regular basis. One day Mildred was put to the test. She was on a community bus coming back from her lunch bunch outing when the bus broke down. The residents on the bus were stranded for over an hour until help arrived. Previously Mildred would not have even attended the social event because of her fear of an incontinence accident. However, this day Mildred felt in control. When they made it back to the community, Mildred dashed off the bus, stopping only briefly to proclaim, "I made it without an accident!" and then rushed into the bathroom. Mildred credits the activity class in helping her with her incontinence problems.

Features of Hold It to Function

The Hold It to Function program features two exercises to strengthen the pelvic muscles. This program also contains eight exercises (both sitting and standing) to strengthen the lower-body muscles.

The main **focus** of Hold It to Function is to improve strength in the pelvic muscles, which will allow older adults to hold their urine for a longer time. This program also helps older adults improve lower-body strength so that they can transfer faster out of a chair or bed and get to the bathroom before an accident occurs.

The **participant** who will benefit from this program

- has frequent incontinence accidents;
- is unable to get to the bathroom in time once an urge to void hits; and
- has poor balance, difficulty walking, and difficulty transferring out of a chair.

The following are **practical benefits** of Hold It to Function:

- It improves lower-body strength so that people can transfer and walk to the bathroom faster before an accident occurs.
- It improves balance so that older adults are less likely to fall.
- It strengthens pelvic floor muscles, so those with incontinence problems can hold urine longer.
- It decreases incontinence accidents.
- It increases participation in social activities because participants are not afraid of having incontinence accidents.

Here are the **guidelines** to follow as you lead this program:

- Offer the Hold It to Function class at least two days per week.
- Participants should perform Kegel exercises two to five times per day outside of class.

- Perform 10 repetitions of each exercise.
- Participants should increase the number of Kegels performed weekly.
- Distribute the door hanger to any person who has problems with bladder control. Make a photocopy of the door hanger on page 126. Cut it out and fold on the solid line that runs down the middle. Laminate it, then cut along the slanted dotted line and around the black circle to enable you to hang it on the resident's bathroom or room door. The door hanger will serve as a reminder to perform the exercises.

This program requires no **equipment.**

Hold It to Function Program Elements

Here are the exercises for the Hold It to Function program. The program guide for Hold It to Function is on page 120, and the page numbers where the description of each exercise will be found are noted after each exercise named in the following lists:

Chat

Talk about successes or problems.

Provide guidelines and support.

Sitting Exercises

Leg extension, page 89

Circle and point, page 91

Pelvic Floor Exercises

Two sets of 5 to 10 Kegels, page 126

Pelvic Floor Exercises

Three sets of 5 to 10 Kegels, page 126

5 to 8 repetitions of leg squeeze, page 89

Standing Exercises

Heel and toe, page 91

Knee raise, page 93

Leg to side and cross, page 94

Leg to back, page 95

Leg curl, page 95

Squats, page 97

Maintaining Hold It to Function Gains

To maintain all of the benefits acquired through the Hold It to Function program, participants should continue performing the Kegel exercises. As participants' confidence to attend more activities increases, encourage them to attend a strength training class, such as Squeeze to Function or Strengthen to Function, to maintain lower-body strength while improving upper-body strength.

MOVE TO FUNCTION

Staying active, in whatever capacity, is an important part of staying healthy. Even older persons with significant physical limitations, including those confined to bed, can benefit from some degree of physical activity. If a person is temporarily or permanently bedridden as a result of injury or illness, other concerns exist. Most people who are unable to get out of bed have difficulty moving around in the bed as well. Changing positions can be difficult, and lying in one position for too long can lead to pressure sores and ulcers. Turning or helping a person

---

Success Story

RISE AND WALK

After suffering a mild stroke and falling and fracturing her hip, Nettie was in bed for months. It became more and more difficult for her to transfer out of bed without assistance from the aides. Once she was out of bed, she relied on a wheelchair to get to the bathroom or go to dinner. Nettie's roommate, Jan, was very active, attending every activity offered at the facility. She especially liked the Squeeze to Function class. Every day Jan would encourage Nettie to get out of bed and exercise. Nettie wouldn't get out of bed because she was so weak she had difficulty transferring from the bed to a chair. She also was afraid of falling. After a while, Nettie saw how much Jan was improving and all the fun she was having. So Nettie decided she wanted to start exercising and get out of her bed. Nettie called the activity director and told her she wanted to start to exercise. The activity director met with Nettie three times per week for the Move to Function activity program. As the activity director was working with Nettie, Jan watched and learned as well. After a few sessions, Jan would work with Nettie on the days the activity director didn't come to their room. Within a month, Nettie was able to get out of bed unassisted and attend the Lift to Function activity program. Jan now volunteers her time to help other residents who are bedridden.

---

turn onto the back or side every two hours can help prevent pressure-related problems.

Range of motion exercises in which a limb is gently moved through its normal movements (for example, bending and straightening the arm at the elbow) can help prevent muscles from becoming tight and joints from becoming stiff. The key is to perform the exercises slowly and to watch and listen for reactions signaling discomfort. Participants should stop doing an exercise if it causes extreme pain.

Features of Move to Function

The Move to Function exercise program can be performed while the participant is in bed. Although all of the exercises can be performed while reclining in bed, the goal is to gradually progress the participant to stand up next to the bed and exercise.

The Move to Function exercise program features 9 upper-body exercises to improve flexibility. Four lower-body exercises are included to increase leg and foot circulation. Finally, eight exercises using small resistance balls (same as those used for Squeeze to Function) improve upper-body strength.

The main **focus** of Move to Function is to improve range of motion so that older adults can perform basic activities by themselves, such as dressing, grooming, and eating. Improving upper-body strength aids in transferring out of bed and sitting up straight in bed.

The **participant** who will benefit from this program

- is bedridden,
- only leaves the bed for meals,
- cannot stand on her own,
- uses a wheelchair for transportation, and
- is unable to perform many activities of daily living such as dressing and bathing.

The following are **practical benefits** of Move to Function:

- It improves upper-body range of motion to perform dressing and grooming.
- It improves upper-body strength for eating and transferring.
- It improves circulation in the lower legs.

Here are the **guidelines** to follow as you lead this program:

- Participants should exercise one to two times per day.
- The goal is to get the participants out of bed to stand to exercise.
- Participants should sit up as straight as possible in bed.
- The back should be flat against a headboard or pillow.
- Participants should perform 10 repetitions of each exercise.

The **equipment** required for this program is two small balls that provide resistance.

Move to Function Program Elements

Here are the exercises for the Move to Function program. The program guide for Move to Function is on page 122, and the page numbers where the description of each exercise can be found are noted after each exercise named in the following lists:

Upper-Body Exercises

Shoulder circles, page 72

Neck stretch, page 72

Arm stretch, page 73

Arm push, page 74

Arm circles, page 74

Back squeeze, page 75

Hugs, page 76

Wrist circles and extensions, page 76

Thumb to finger, page 76

Lower-Body Exercises

Circle and point, page 91

Scrunch and wiggle, page 106

Knee raise, page 93

Leg to side and cross, page 94

Ball Exercises

Ball squeeze, page 80

Roll and press, page 80

Top and bottom press, page 81

Shoulder squeeze, page 81

Lateral raise, page 83

One-arm row, page 84

Biceps curl, page 85

Wiper, page 85

Maintaining Move to Function Gains

Encourage participants at all times to sit up and get out of bed. Once they can get out of bed, encourage them to participate in the Lift to Function program.

REMEMBER TO FUNCTION

People with dementia may need extra attention in order to learn how to perform various exercises. They also may require more time to perform the exercises than participants without dementia require. To reduce distraction and anxiety caused by the extra attention and the slowdown in the class, fitness instructors should offer a separate class for people with dementia.

Success Story

GOTTA KEEP MOVING!

Rose was a participant in the Remember to Function program. Although she enjoyed being in class and participating in all of the activities, she could never recall that she had exercised. One night at 3:00 a.m., Rose was wandering around the hallway. The night nurse stopped and asked Rose where she was going. Rose replied, "I'm going to exercise."

Features of Remember to Function

The Remember to Function exercise program has been developed specifically for people with dementia. It contains eight simple exercises using large and small balls to improve upper-body strength, range of motion, and performance of daily activities. Four leg exercises are included to improve lower-body strength as well as balance. Regular participation in the Remember to Function program can help older adults decrease or manage behavioral disturbances common in people with dementia, such as wandering, outbursts, and agitation.

The main **focus** of Remember to Function is to provide structure in participants' daily routines and maintain their quality of life for as long as possible. People with dementia can successfully perform these exercises and achieve a sense of accomplishment.

The **participant** who will benefit from this program has

- dementia or Alzheimer's disease,
- memory-related problems,
- loss of cognitive functions, or
- behavioral disturbances (wandering, agitation).

The following are **practical benefits** of Remember to Function:

- It decreases wandering, agitation, and physical and verbal outbursts.
- It improves sleep patterns.
- It improves balance and decreases falls.
- It allows older adults to perform daily activities by themselves.
- It provides structure to daily routines.
- It improves cognitive capacity.
- It increases energy expenditure.

Here are the **guidelines** to follow as you lead this program:

- Offer a separate class just for people with dementia. Limit the class to 15 participants.
- Enlist caregivers who are familiar with the participants to help gather them for class and help them exercise.
- To avoid unnecessary distraction, try to have all participants seated in class before you start the exercises.
- Perform exercises daily, preferably at the same time each day. Make exercise a positive aspect of their daily routines.
- Stand or sit in front of the participants so that they can see you perform the exercises.
- Perform 10 repetitions of each exercise unless otherwise stated. Encourage participants to count along with you.
- Provide constant verbal and visual cues to describe how to perform each exercise (for example, "Squeeze the lemon").
- Encourage active participation rather than perfection. (As long as participants are not injuring themselves, do not repeatedly attempt to change their technique if they are performing the exercise incorrectly.)
- Use a mirror image while performing the exercises so that participants can follow along with few complications. Participants will be able to follow you better if you are lifting the arm on the same side as they are if you are facing them.
- Touch the arm or leg that should be lifted to help them identify their right or left body parts.
- Remember, participants will mimic everything you do. Be careful in your actions.
- Begin each exercise session with a short chat time, approximately five minutes. Talk about the weather, the date, and the season.
- If participants are reluctant to exercise, start with an exercise they particularly enjoy.

The following is the **equipment** required for this program:

- Large play balls
- Small balls that provide resistance

Remember to Function Program Elements

Here are the exercises for the Remember to Function program. The program guide for Remember to Function is on page 124, and the page numbers where the description of each exercise can be found are noted after each exercise named in the following lists:

Maintaining Remember to Function Gains

To get the most from the Remember to Function program, older adults should participate in the program on a daily basis.

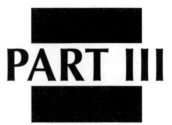

PART III

Exercise Instructions and Program Guides

Information on how to perform each exercise correctly as well as program guides to facilitate leading programs are presented in part III. Chapter 6 provides exercise illustrations, instructions, and modifications for all the exercises featured in *Functional Fitness for Older Adults*. Some of the illustrations for upper-body exercises feature participants using dumbbells. You can use dumbbells, balls, or no weights to perform these exercises. The illustrations for lower-body exercises feature participants using ankle weights. Again, participants also can perform these exercises without weights. To help you lead the exercise programs effectively, chapter 7 includes program guides to summarize each program. You may copy, enlarge, and laminate these charts. When you are conducting each program, select the appropriate chart and lay it on the floor in front of you as a handy reminder of the proper order of and technique for the exercises.

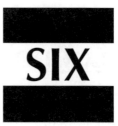

SIX

Exercise Instructions

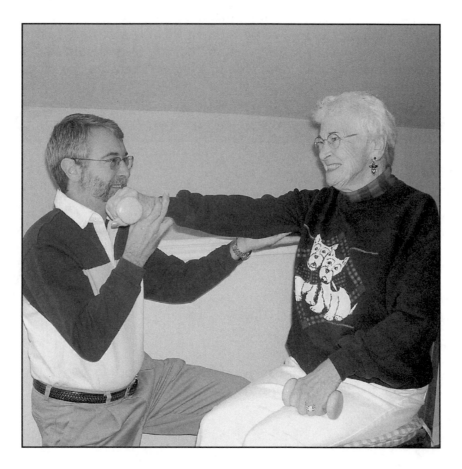

To ensure the safety of your participants, make sure they do the exercises correctly. This chapter includes information on the functional purpose of the exercise, the muscles used to perform the exercise, how to perform the exercise, and adaptations to the exercise for those people who have difficulty performing the exercise as shown. For example, an older adult with poor balance may not want to stand to perform the leg exercises. Seated adaptations are provided so that a person with poor balance can perform the exercise with the group while seated. Many of the exercises also include suggestions to make the exercise into a gamelike activity rather than simply a boring calisthenic experience. These ideas may help you get started, but you can also use your own ideas to keep your participants engaged. Finally, some of the exercises have an "Additional Notes" section that includes miscellaneous information on the exercise.

WARM-UP AND COOL-DOWN EXERCISES

Be sure to include adequate warm-up periods in your activity program, regardless of the overall goal of the program. Warming up before performing the exercises in the activity program gradually increases circulation and heart rate and prepares the body for movement that will occur during the program. The following are warm-up exercises for all of the activity programs. You can also use some of these warm-up exercises during the cool-down period. Participants should do all warm-up and cool-down exercises in a slow and controlled manner for safety and for optimal muscle strengthening. (Performing exercises fast does not strengthen muscles as well as performing them slowly does.) Encourage participants to stretch as far as they can and hold it. They should stretch only to the point of minimal pain. Walk around the class to ensure participants are stretching properly.

SHOULDER CIRCLES

Functional Purpose

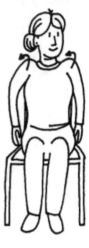

- Improving range of motion in the shoulders and upper-back.
- Warming up to prevent injury while exercising.

Muscles Worked

- Shoulders (deltoids)
- Upper back (trapezius)

Instructions

- Slowly circle the shoulders backward five times. Repeat circling the shoulders forward five times.

Adaptations

- Circle one shoulder at a time.

For Those Needing More of a Challenge

- Hold weights in hands with arms extended down to the floor.

Ideas for Fun

- Pretend you are rowing a boat. Row forward and backward.

NECK STRETCH

Functional Purpose

- Stretching to increase flexibility.
- Increasing range of motion in the neck area when turning side to side and down.

Muscles Worked

- Neck (sternocleidomastoid)

Instructions

- Slowly turn head over right shoulder. Hold. Return to center. Slowly lower chin to chest. Hold. Slowly turn head over left shoulder. Hold. Repeat series three times.

Adaptations

- Turn head only to the point of mild pain. Hold for 10 seconds.

Ideas for Fun

- Imagine someone is behind you. Turn to the left to see who it is. Can't see them? Turn to the right.
- Pretend you are backing out of the driveway and you need to see if the dog is in the way.

Additional Notes

- Never stretch the head toward the back. This does not stretch any muscles and could be harmful for those participants with osteoporosis or claudications in the neck.

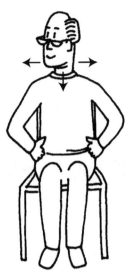

ARM STRETCH

Functional Purpose

- Increasing range of motion in the arms, shoulders, and back.
- Warming up to prevent injury while exercising.
- Stretching shoulder and arm muscles to ease transfer out of a bed or chair.

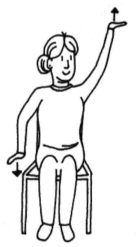

Muscles Worked

- Shoulders (deltoids)
- Upper back (trapezius)
- Lower back (latissimus dorsi, erector spinae)

Instructions

- Push the right palm up toward the ceiling. Push the left palm down toward the floor. Hold. Bring both arms to front of chest. Switch arms and hold. Repeat series three times.

Adaptations

- Raise arm toward the ceiling as high as possible. If a participant has limited range of motion because of a stroke or surgery, encourage him to raise his arm as high as possible. Every day he should be able to raise it a little bit farther. The same principle applies to the arm pushing down to the floor.

Ideas for Fun

- Reach up high and grab a star.
- Push down toward the ground to stop the gopher from coming out of his hole.

ARM PUSH

Functional Purpose

- Increasing range of motion in the arms, shoulders, and back.
- Warming up to prevent injury while exercising.

Muscles Worked

- Shoulders (deltoids)
- Upper back (trapezius)
- Lower back (latissimus dorsi, erector spinae)

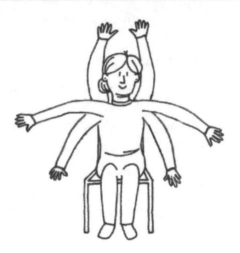

Instructions

- Stretch both arms up toward the ceiling. Hold. Stretch both arms out to the side. Hold. Stretch both arms down toward the floor. Hold. Repeat series three times.

Adaptations

- If a participant has limited range of motion because of a stroke or surgery, encourage her to raise her arms as high as possible. Every day she should be able to raise them a little bit farther. The same principle applies to the arms pushing out to the side and down to the floor.

Ideas for Fun

- Push up to hold up the ceiling. Push out to the side as though you were pushing the walls of a room out to make it larger. Push down.

ARM CIRCLES

Functional Purpose

- Improving range of motion in the shoulders and upper back.
- Warming up to prevent injury while exercising.
- Increasing range of motion to be able to reach items on a shelf.

Muscles Worked

- Shoulders (deltoids)

Instructions

- Begin by making small circles with the right arm. Gradually increase the size until you make full circles. Stop. Repeat, circling in the opposite direction. Repeat circles in both directions with the left arm.

For Those Needing More of a Challenge

- Hold a one- to two-pound weight.

Ideas for Fun

- Circle in a clockwise or counterclockwise position, stopping at different times.

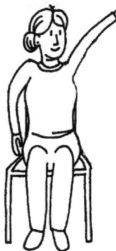

BACK SQUEEZE

Functional Purpose

- Improving range of motion in the shoulders and upper back.
- Warming up to prevent injury while exercising.
- Pushing shoulders back for good posture.

Muscles Worked

- Upper back (trapezius)
- Lower back (latissimus dorsi)

Instructions

- Pull elbows back behind the body. Squeeze shoulder blades together. Hold. Repeat three to five times.

Adaptations

- Participants with newly implanted pacemakers or those who have had heart surgery should not perform this exercise until they receive clearance from their physicians.

Ideas for Fun

- Squeeze the shoulders back to try to pop open the buttons on your shirt.

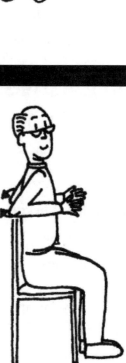

HUGS

Functional Purpose

- Improving range of motion in upper back.
- Warming up to prevent injury while exercising.

Muscles Worked

- Lower back (latissimus dorsi)
- Shoulders (deltoids)

Instructions

- Cross arms in front of body and hug yourself. Switch arms and hug. Repeat hugs three to five times.

Ideas for Fun

- Give yourself a hug and a pat on the back.

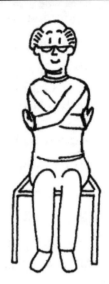

WRIST CIRCLES AND EXTENSIONS

Functional Purpose

- Increasing range of motion in the wrists and fingers to aid in performing fine motor movements such as opening jars and buttoning blouses.

Muscles Worked

- Wrist muscles

Instructions

- Circle wrists outward 10 times. Reverse, circling wrists inward 10 times. Extend fingers out, spreading them as far apart as possible. Relax. Repeat 5 times.

Ideas for Fun

- Pretend you are conducting an orchestra.

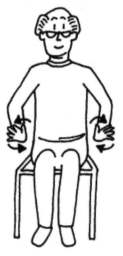

THUMB TO FINGER

Functional Purpose

- Increasing range of motion in the fingers to aid in performing fine motor movements such as opening jars and buttoning blouses.
- Decreasing arthritis flare-ups.

Muscles Worked

- Muscles in fingers and hands

Instructions

- Slowly touch the thumb to each finger. Reverse directions and repeat. Repeat series 10 times.

Ideas for Fun

- Pretend you are playing the piano.

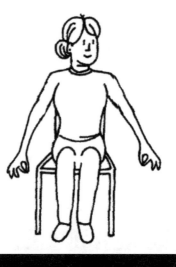

QUADRICEPS STRETCH

Functional Purpose

- Warming up to prevent injury while exercising.
- Stretching to increase flexibility and prevent injury during walking and stair climbing.

Muscles Worked

- Thighs (quadriceps)

Instructions

- With the left hand holding onto the chair, grab the right ankle with the right hand. Slowly pull the heel up toward the buttocks. The right knee should be close to the left knee. Hold for 10 seconds. Relax. Repeat, stretching the right leg two or three times before stretching the left leg.

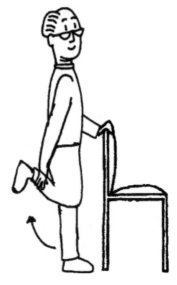

Ideas for Fun

- Pretend you are a pink flamingo standing on one leg.

Additional Notes

- Make sure the knee of the leg being stretched is close to the other knee.

CALF STRETCH

Functional Purpose

- Warming up to prevent injury while exercising.
- Stretching to increase flexibility and prevent injury during walking and stair climbing.

Muscles Worked

- Calves (gastrocnemius)

Instructions

- Holding on to the back of a chair, slowly extend the right leg back. Push the heel to the floor and hold for 10 seconds. Switch legs and repeat the stretch on the left leg. Repeat series three times.

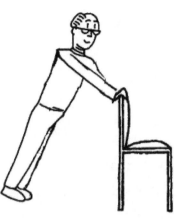

DEEP BREATHING

Functional Purpose

- Inhaling large breaths to expand the rib cage and get more air to the lungs.

Muscles Worked

- Diaphragm

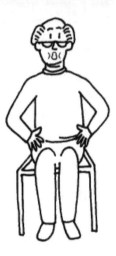

Instructions

- Slowly take a deep breath in through the nose. Slowly exhale through the mouth. Repeat deep breathing three to five times.

Additional Notes

- Breathing should be slow. Fast breathing may cause dizziness.

UPPER-BODY EXERCISES

These exercises can improve the upper-body strength of older adults. You can incorporate resistance into the following exercises through the use of accessories such as small balls, large balls, and dumbbells. Use a mirror image while conducting the upper-body exercises. Participants will be able to follow you better if you are lifting the arm on the same side as they are if you are facing them. Have your class count as you perform the exercises.

ARM PRESS AND PULL

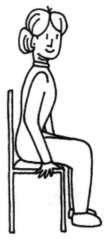

Functional Purpose

- Strengthening shoulder and arm muscles to ease the transfer out of a bed or chair.

Muscles Worked

- Chest (pectorals)
- Shoulders (deltoids)
- Front of arms (biceps)

Instructions

- Sit at the edge of a chair and slowly press down on the edge, lifting the body slightly upward. Hold for three seconds. Relax. Grab underneath the chair and pull up. Hold for three seconds. Repeat series five times.

CHAIR LIFT

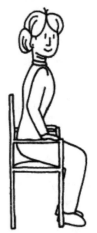

Functional Purpose

- Strengthening shoulder and arm muscles to ease the transfer out of a bed or chair.

Muscles Worked

- Chest (pectorals)
- Shoulders (deltoids)
- Front of arms (biceps)

Instructions

- Place hands on arms of the chair next to sides. Slowly push down until the arms are extended and the buttocks are off the chair. Hold for three seconds. Slowly lower to seated position. Repeat five times.

Adaptations

- If chairs do not have arms, perform 10 wall push-ups.

BALL SQUEEZE

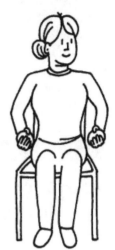

Functional Purpose

- Strengthening wrist and forearm muscles to improve grip strength.

Muscles Worked

- Wrists
- Forearms

Instructions

- Place a small ball in each hand. Slowly squeeze the balls, then release. Squeeze balls 20 times.

Adaptations

- Participants with rheumatoid arthritis should not perform the ball squeeze.

Ideas for Fun

- Squeeze the balls as if you are squeezing lemons to make lemonade.

SIDE PRESS

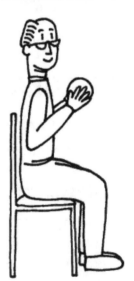

Functional Purpose

- Strengthening chest and shoulder muscles to aid in driving, yard work, and housework.

Muscles Worked

- Chest (pectorals)
- Shoulders (deltoids)

Instructions

- Place a ball between palms in front of the chest. Press hands toward each other and squeeze the chest muscles. Hold for three counts. Relax. Repeat.

ROLL AND PRESS

Functional Purpose

- Strengthening chest muscles to lift and carry items.
- Improving hand coordination.

Muscles Worked

- Chest (pectorals)
- Shoulders (deltoids)
- Front of arms (biceps)

Instructions

- Place a ball between palms in front of the chest. Roll the ball eight times. Stop rolling and press hands toward each other to squeeze the chest muscles. Hold for three counts. Relax. Repeat.

Ideas for Fun

- We are going to make bread. Roll the ball as though you are rolling a ball of dough. Now squeeze the dough. Roll again.

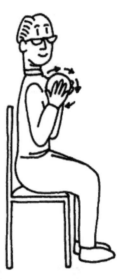

TOP AND BOTTOM PRESS

Functional Purpose

- Strengthening chest, arm, and back muscles to transfer, prepare meals, or garden.

Muscles Worked

- Chest (pectorals)
- Upper back (trapezius)

Instructions

- Place one hand on top and the other hand below the ball. Slowly press the ball together between the hands. Hold. Relax. Repeat ball press eight times, then switch hand position.

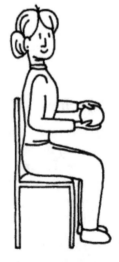

SHOULDER SQUEEZE

Functional Purpose

- Strengthening shoulder and arm muscles to help with self-care activities and wheelchair mobility.

Muscles Worked

- Shoulders (deltoids)
- Front of arms (biceps)

Instructions

- Place a ball in each hand and place the hands on the front of the shoulders. Slowly squeeze the balls into the shoulders. Relax and repeat.

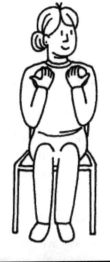

SHOULDER PRESS

Functional Purpose

- Strengthening shoulder and back muscles to help with transferring out of a chair or bed.

Muscles Worked

- Shoulders (deltoids)
- Upper back (trapezius)

Instructions

- Start with hands on knees, palms facing down. Place the right hand on the shoulder, palm facing out. Slowly extend the right hand up toward the ceiling. Hold. Slowly lower the hand back to the shoulder. Repeat, lifting the right hand for the desired number of repetitions before lifting the left hand.

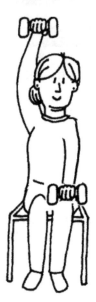

Adaptations

- Participants who have limited range of motion because of a stroke or surgery should raise the arm up as high as possible without causing extreme pain. Using no dumbbell or a lighter dumbbell than the one used for the good arm is recommended.

FRONT RAISE

Functional Purpose

- Strengthening shoulders to help perform grooming and reaching.

Muscles Worked

- Shoulders (deltoids)
- Top of chest (pectorals)

Instructions

- Place the hands on the knees, palms facing down. Slowly raise the right hand straight in front of the body until it reaches shoulder level. Hold. Slowly lower hand to knee. Repeat, lifting the right arm for the desired number of repetitions before lifting the left arm. Do not raise the dumbbells past shoulder level.

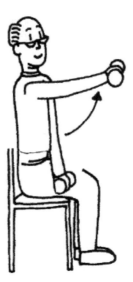

Adaptations

- Participants who have limited range of motion because of a stroke or surgery should raise the arm up as high as possible without causing extreme pain. Using no dumbbell or a lighter dumbbell than the one used for the good arm is recommended.

For Those Needing More of a Challenge

- Use dumbbells or balls with these exercises.

LATERAL RAISE

Functional Purpose

- Strengthening shoulders and upper back to help lift and carry items and improve posture.
- Being able to throw a ball to a dog.

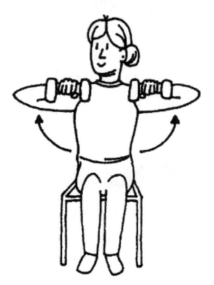

Muscles Worked

- Shoulders (deltoids)
- Upper back (trapezius)

Instructions

- Bend arms at a 90 degree angle next to sides with palms facing inward. Swing the arms up until they are parallel to the floor. Slowly lower arms to starting position. Repeat.

Adaptations

- If using balls, squeeze the balls before lifting the arms.
- Participants who have limited range of motion because of a stroke or surgery should raise the arms up as high as possible without causing extreme pain. Using no dumbbell or a lighter dumbbell than the one used for the good arm is recommended.

Ideas for Fun

- Act like a chicken and raise your wings.

UPRIGHT ROW

Functional Purpose

- Strengthening upper-back muscles to help lift heavy items and pull on pants.

Muscles Worked

- Shoulders (deltoids)
- Upper back (trapezius)

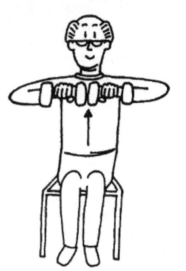

Instructions

- Place both hands down in front of the thighs, palms facing toward the thighs. Keeping hands together and close to the body, slowly raise hands toward the chin by bending the elbows. Hold. Return to the starting position. Repeat.

Adaptations

- You can use balls or light dumbbells. If using balls, squeeze the balls before lifting the arms.
- Participants who have limited range of motion because of a stroke or surgery should raise the arms up as high as possible without causing extreme pain. Using no dumbbell or a lighter dumbbell than the one used for the good arm is recommended.

Ideas for Fun

- Raise the weights as if you are washing clothes on a washboard.

ONE-ARM ROW

Functional Purpose

- Strengthening back muscles to improve posture and balance.

Muscles Worked

- Back (latissimus dorsi)
- Upper back (trapezius)
- Front of arms (biceps)

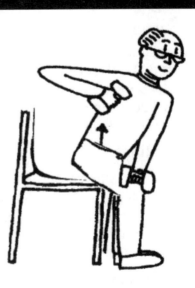

Instructions

- Scoot to the edge of the chair and lean forward. Extend the right arm down toward the floor with the palm facing inward. Slowly raise the hand up toward the armpit. Keep the hand close to the body. Lower the hand to the starting position. Repeat, lifting the right hand for the desired number of repetitions before lifting the left hand.

Adaptations

- You can use dumbbells or balls with these exercises. If using balls, squeeze the balls before lifting the arms.
- Participants who have limited range of motion because of a stroke or surgery should raise the arm up as high as possible without causing extreme pain. Using no dumbbell or a lighter dumbbell than used for the good arm is recommended.

BICEPS CURL

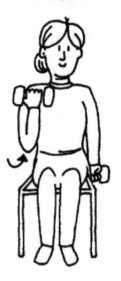

Functional Purpose

- Strengthening biceps muscles used in activities such as fishing, cooking, and yard work.

Muscles Worked

- Front of arms (biceps)

Instructions

- Place hands on thighs, palms facing up. Slowly lift the right hand to the shoulder. Slowly lower hand to thigh. Repeat, lifting the right hand before lifting the left hand.

Adaptations

- If using balls, squeeze the balls before lifting the arms.
- Participants who have limited range of motion because of a stroke or surgery should raise the arm up as high as possible without causing extreme pain. Using no dumbbell or a lighter dumbbell than used in the good arm is recommended.

Ideas for Fun

- Do the Popeye exercise: Lift the can of spinach.

WIPER

Functional Purpose

- Strengthening back of arm to help transfer out of a chair.
- Tightening underarm area.

Muscles Worked

- Back of arms (triceps)

Instructions

- Point right elbow out to the side of the body while placing right hand on edge of chest. Keeping the elbow stationary, slowly extend hand out to the side so that arm forms a straight line. (Arm should be parallel to the floor.) Slowly return hand to starting position. Repeat, extending the right arm for the desired number of repetitions before extending the left arm.

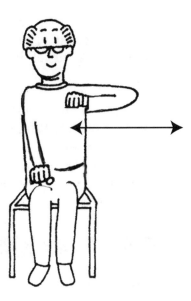

Adaptations

- If using balls, squeeze the balls before lifting the arms.
- Participants who have limited range of motion because of a stroke or surgery should raise the arm up as high as possible without causing extreme pain. Using no dumbbell or a lighter dumbbell than used for the good arm is recommended.

Ideas for Fun

- Pretend you are a windshield wiper on a car.

TRICEPS EXTENSION

Functional Purpose

- Strengthening back of arm to help transfer out of a chair.
- Tightening underarm area.

Muscles Worked

- Back of arms (triceps)

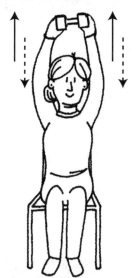

Instructions

- Hold one ball or dumbbell with both hands. Raise arms overhead. Slowly lower hands behind head, keeping elbows pointed toward the ceiling. Extend hands back toward ceiling. Repeat.

Adaptations

- Place dumbbell in front of chest. Slowly push down toward thighs.
- You can use dumbbells or balls with these exercises. If using a ball, squeeze the ball before lowering the arms.
- Participants who have limited range of motion because of a stroke or surgery should raise the arms up as high as possible without causing extreme pain. Using no dumbbell or a lighter dumbbell than the one used for the good arm is recommended.

ABDOMINAL EXERCISES

Strong abdominal muscles are important for maintaining good posture and balance and for performing many daily activities. In some cases, weak abdominal muscles are associated with low back pain.

REVERSE CURL

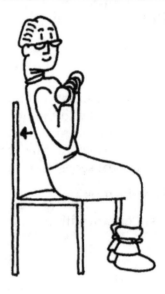

Functional Purpose

- Strengthening abdominal muscles for improved posture and balance and less back pain.

Muscles Worked

- Abdominals
- Lower back (erector spinae)

Instructions

- Sit on edge of chair. Place both hands on chest. Slowly lean back without touching the back of the chair. Hold for three seconds. Return to starting position. Repeat.

Ideas for Fun

- Lean back in your chair as if you were spying on your neighbor.

ABDOMINAL TWIST

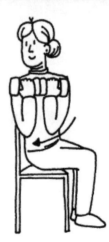

Functional Purpose

- Strengthening sides of the body for improved posture and balance.

Muscles Worked

- Sides (obliques)
- Abdominals

Instructions

- Sit on edge of chair or stand. Begin with the hands resting on the collarbone. Twist toward the right. Hold. Return to the center, then twist toward the left. Repeat.

Adaptations

- Use dumbbells or balls with these exercises.

SIDE BENDS

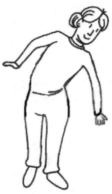

Functional Purpose

- Stretching the sides of the body for improved flexibility.
- Increasing ability to reach down and pick an object up off the floor.

Muscles Worked

- Sides (obliques)

Instructions

- Hold arms straight down next to the sides. Slowly bend over to the right side. Hold for three seconds. Slowly return to the upright standing position. Slowly bend over to the left side. Hold for three seconds. Slowly return to the upright standing position. Repeat series three times.

Adaptations

- Perform with or without dumbbells.

LOWER-BODY SITTING EXERCISES

The following exercises improve lower-body strength. Improvement in lower-body strength can help older adults perform daily activities such as walking, climbing stairs, getting down on the floor to play with grandchildren, and playing sports such as golf. Leg strength also improves balance and decreases the risk for falls. Resistance can be incorporated into these exercises through the use of ankle weights. Use a mirror image while conducting each lower-body exercise. Participants will be able to follow you better if you are lifting the leg on the same side as they are if you are facing them. Have your class count as you perform the exercises.

LEG SQUEEZE

Functional Purpose

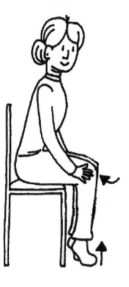

- Strengthening leg muscles to get to the bathroom faster once an urge to void hits.
- Strengthening pelvic floor muscles to hold urine longer without having an accident.

Muscles Worked

- Pelvic floor muscles
- Buttocks (gluteals)
- Thighs (quadriceps)

Instructions

- Rise up on the toes. Squeeze the knees, thighs, and buttock muscles together. Hold for three counts. Relax. Repeat.

Adaptations

- Perform with or without a ball

For Those Needing More of a Challenge

- Place a ball between knees while squeezing.

LEG EXTENSION

Functional Purpose

- Strengthening thigh muscles to improve walking, gait speed, and skill in rising from a chair.
- Older adults will be able to climb stairs to tuck their grandchildren into bed.

Muscles Worked

- Thighs (quadriceps)

Instructions

- Sitting up straight in a chair, slowly extend the right foot out. Hold. Slowly lower the foot to the floor. Repeat, lifting the right foot for the desired number of repetitions before lifting the left foot.

For Those Needing More of a Challenge

- Wear ankle weights.

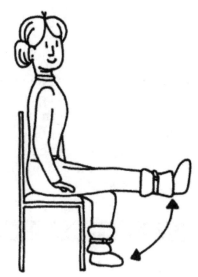

LOWER-BODY STANDING EXERCISES AND SEATED MODIFICATIONS

The following exercises improve lower-body strength, which can help older adults perform daily activities such as walking, climbing stairs, getting down on the floor to play with grandchildren, and playing sports such as golf. Leg strength also improves balance and decreases the risk for falls. Resistance can be incorporated into these exercises through the use of ankle weights. Modifications to each exercise are provided for those participants who might not be able to stand to perform the exercises. Performing the seated exercises will enable older adults to exercise the same muscle groups as if they were standing up.

CIRCLE AND POINT

Functional Purpose

- Improving strength and circulation in the ankles, allowing for better reaction time from swaying or tripping.
- Improving balance.

Muscles Worked

- Ankles
- Calves (gastrocnemius)
- Shins (soleus)

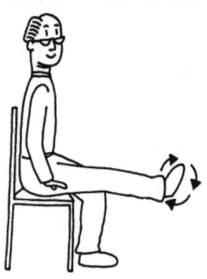

Instructions

- Extend right foot out and circle the ankle outward. Repeat, circling the ankle inward. Point the toes up toward the ceiling and down toward the floor. Repeat circles and points with the left foot.

Adaptations

- Perform with or without ankle weights.

For Those Needing More of a Challenge

- Wear ankle weights.

HEEL AND TOE STANDING, HEEL AND TOE SITTING

Functional Purpose

- Strengthening the calf and ankle muscles to improve mobility and balance, which will decrease the risk of falls.

Muscles Worked

- Calves (gastrocnemius)
- Shins (soleus)
- Ankles

Instructions

- Hold onto the back of a chair. Stand with feet close together. Maintaining good posture, slowly raise up on the toes. Hold. Slowly rock back on the heels. Hold. Repeat.

Adaptations

- While sitting, rise up on the toes. Hold. Slowly rock back on the heels. Repeat.
- Can be performed with or without ankle weights.

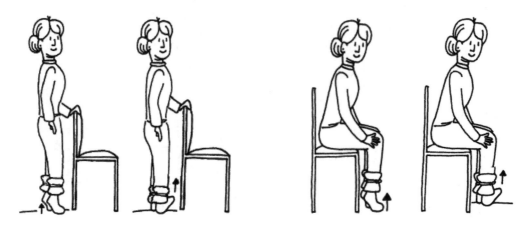

For Those Needing More of a Challenge

- Wear ankle weights.

Ideas for Fun

- Raise up on the toes like you are looking over a fence. Roll back on the heels like a rocking chair.

Additional Notes

- Participants with peripheral vascular disease may experience leg pain while performing this exercise. Once pain occurs, have them stop until the pain subsides.

KNEE RAISE STANDING, KNEE RAISE SITTING

Functional Purpose

- Strengthening thigh muscles to improve mobility and balance.
- Being able to walk and stand longer to shop or go out to lunch.

Muscles Worked

- Thighs (quadriceps)
- Hips (fascia latae)

Instructions

- Stand with feet shoulder-width apart. Maintaining good posture, slowly raise the right knee. Hold. Slowly lower foot to floor. Repeat, lifting the right knee for the desired number of repetitions before lifting the left knee.

Adaptations

- While sitting or lying in the bed, raise knee. Hold. Lower to floor. Repeat.
- Perform with or without ankle weights.

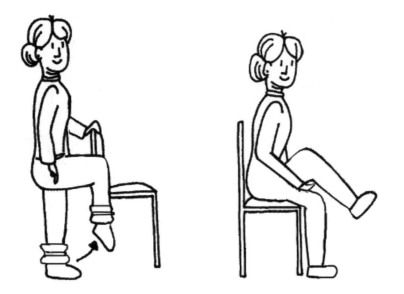

For Those Needing More of a Challenge

- Wear ankle weights.

LEG TO SIDE AND CROSS STANDING, LEG TO SIDE AND CROSS SITTING

Functional Purpose

- Strengthening hip muscles to help with balance and rising from a chair.
- Improving step height so that fewer trips occur.

Muscles Worked

- Hips (abductors)
- Inner thighs (adductors)

Instructions

- Stand with feet shoulder-width apart. Keeping back straight, slowly raise the right leg out to the side away from the body (approximately one foot). Hold. Slowly cross leg in front of body, then return to starting position. Repeat, lifting the right leg for the desired number of repetitions before lifting the left leg.

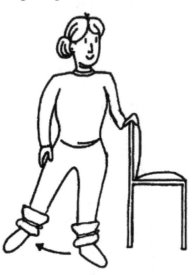 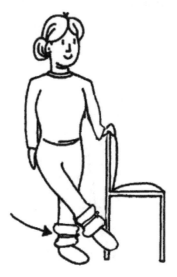

Adaptations

- While sitting or lying in the bed, extend the right leg out in front. Slowly swing the leg out to the side. Hold. Cross leg over knee. Return to starting position. Repeat, lifting the right leg for the desired number of repetitions before lifting the left leg.

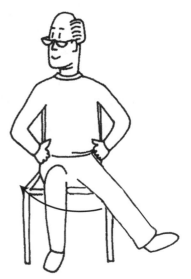

For Those Needing More of a Challenge

- Wear ankle weights.

Additional Notes

- Individuals with dementia have difficulty crossing the leg in front of the body. Therefore, use only the leg to side part of this exercise with this group.

LEG TO BACK STANDING, LEG TO BACK SITTING

Functional Purpose

- Strengthening back of leg to be able to kneel down and get up.

Muscles Worked

- Back of thighs (hamstrings)

Instructions

- Stand with feet close together. Keeping the legs straight, slowly extend the right leg back off the floor (approximately one foot). As you lift the leg, squeeze the buttock muscles together. Hold. Slowly lower the leg until the foot is on the floor. Repeat, lifting the right leg for the desired number of repetitions before lifting the left leg.

- If performing while sitting, slowly curl leg under chair. Hold. Bring back to starting position. Repeat, lifting the right leg for the desired number of repetitions before lifting the left leg.

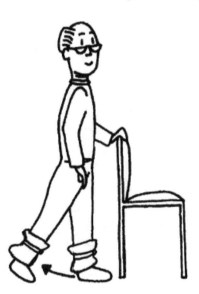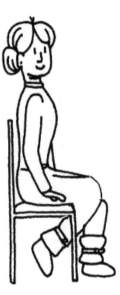

Adaptations

- Perform with or without ankle weights.

For Those Needing More of a Challenge

- Wear ankle weights.

LEG CURL STANDING, LEG CURL SITTING

Functional Purpose

- Strengthening back of leg to be able to kneel down and get up.

Muscles Worked

- Back of thighs (hamstrings)

Instructions

- Stand with feet close together. Maintaining good posture, slowly raise the heel toward the buttocks until the shin is parallel to the floor. Hold. Slowly lower toes to the floor. Repeat, lifting the right foot for the desired number of repetitions before lifting the left foot.
- If performing while sitting, slowly curl leg under chair. Hold. Bring back to starting position. Repeat.

Adaptations

- Perform with or without ankle weights

Additional Notes

- Participants with peripheral vascular disease may experience leg pain while performing this exercise. If pain occurs, have them stop until the pain subsides.

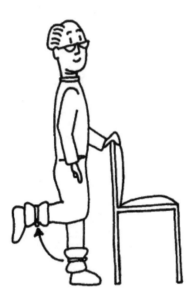 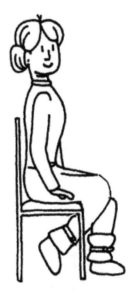

LOWER-BODY STANDING EXERCISES

These exercises can improve the lower-body strength of older adults if performed on a regular basis. Improving lower-body strength will help improve gait and mobility, balance, stair climbing, and transferring in and out of car, bed, or chair. Wear ankle weights to increase the resistance of each exercise.

SQUATS STANDING, SQUATS SITTING

Functional Purpose

- Strengthening leg and buttock muscles to help with walking, balance, and stair climbing.

Muscles Worked

- Thighs (quadriceps)
- Back of thighs (hamstrings)
- Buttocks (gluteals)

Instructions

- Stand with feet shoulder-width apart. With hands on hips and back straight, bend both knees into a squatting position until the knees form a 45-degree angle to the floor. (The knees should not extend past the toes, and the weight of the body should be pressed over the heels.) Slowly stand up straight before repeating.
- If performing while sitting, raise toes off floor. Lean forward and press weight through the heels. Hold for three seconds. Sit back up. Repeat.

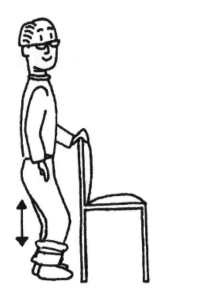 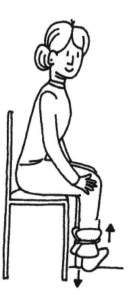

Adaptations

- Perform with or without ankle weights.

Additional Notes

- Participants with peripheral vascular disease may experience leg pain while performing this exercise. If pain occurs, have them stop until the pain subsides.

CHAIR STAND

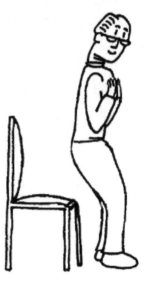

Functional Purpose

- Strengthening leg and buttock muscles to transfer out of a chair or car.

Muscles Worked

- Thighs (quadriceps)
- Back of thighs (hamstrings)
- Buttocks (gluteals)

Instructions

- Place both feet flat on the floor. Cross arms over chest and stand up without the use of the hands. Slowly sit back down to the count of three. Alternate standing up fast and slow. Repeat chair stands five to eight times.

For Those Needing More of a Challenge

- When sitting back down, don't touch the seat.

MARCHING

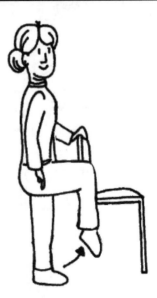

Functional Purpose

- Increasing flexibility of the lower body to climb stairs and to get in and out of the bathtub or car.

Muscles Worked

- Thighs (quadriceps)
- Back of thighs (hamstrings)
- Calves (gastrocnemius)
- Buttocks (gluteals)

Instructions

- Raise knees up in a marching fashion. March fast and slow. March for one to two minutes, rest, then repeat.

Ideas for Fun

- Play marching music.

Additional Notes

- Participants with peripheral vascular disease may experience leg pain while performing this exercise. If pain occurs, have them stop until the pain subsides.

STAIR STEPPING

Functional Purpose

- Strengthening leg and buttock muscles to help with getting out of a chair, walking, mobility, and stair climbing.

Muscles Worked

- Thighs (quadriceps)
- Back of thighs (hamstrings)
- Buttocks (gluteals)

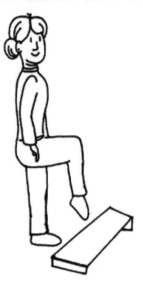

Instructions

- Maintain good posture while stepping. Lean slightly forward while stepping up. Place the entire foot on the center of the step when stepping up. Step ball to heel. Place the whole foot on the floor when stepping down. Step ball to heel.

For Those Needing More of a Challenge

- Increase the step height.

Additional Notes

- Participants with peripheral vascular disease may experience leg pain while performing this exercise. If pain occurs, have them stop until the pain subsides.

INDIVIDUAL BALANCE EXERCISES

The following activities improve standing and seated balance, which will decrease the fear of falling as well as the number of falls in older adults. Improved balance will also increase socialization and participation in activities because participants won't be afraid to walk to an activity. Make this class fun while stressing the importance of improving balance. These exercises can be performed individually or in a group setting.

3-STANCE

Instructions

- Perform the following balance stances for 10 to 20 seconds. Maintain good posture by standing up straight and tightening the abdominal muscles. (Keep a chair nearby for support, but encourage your participants not to hold onto the chair.) Stand in each position with the eyes open, then closed.
- The three positions are 1) feet together, 2) feet semi-tandem (one foot slightly ahead of the other), and 3) feet tandem (one foot directly in front of the other).

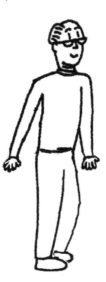 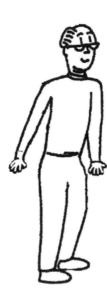 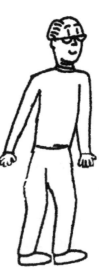

Feet together   **Semi-tandem**   **Tandem**

FOOT STAND

Instructions

- Stand with feet shoulder-width apart. Slowly place the right toes on the left foot. Hold for 5 to 10 seconds. Place the right foot back on the floor. Repeat by placing the left toes on the right foot. Repeat series three to five times.

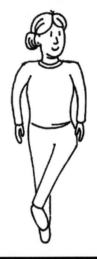

STEP RIGHT AND LEFT

Instructions

- Step sideways in the following pattern: right, left, right, left, right, left. Repeat series going in the opposite direction. Repeat series three to five times.

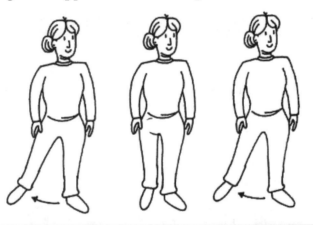

BALL PASS

Instructions

- Pass a ball around the head, chest, wrist, and knees. Repeat by passing the ball in the opposite direction. Repeat series three to five times.

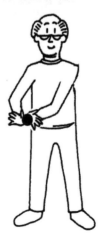

TANDEM WALK

Instructions

- Walk heel to toe for 10 feet. (Use a rail or wall for support.) Walk backward, toe to heel, for 10 feet. Repeat series three to five times.

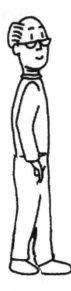

FOOT ALPHABET

Instructions

- Spell the alphabet with the right foot, then with the left foot.

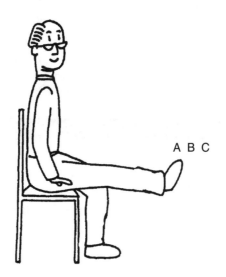

GROUP BALANCE EXERCISES STANDING IN A LINE

Be sure that participants are standing close enough to one another to perform the exercises safely.

OVERHEAD BALL PASS

Instructions

- Pass a ball overhead to the person behind you. Once the ball has reached the end of the line, pass the ball overhead in a forward manner. Repeat two to three times.

BALL PASS BETWEEN LEGS

Instructions

- Pass the ball between the legs to the person behind you. Once the ball has reached the end of the line, pass the ball forward between the legs. Repeat two to three times.

ALTERNATE HEAD AND LEGS

Instructions

- Start by passing a ball overhead to the person behind you. That person then passes the ball between his legs to the person behind him. Once the ball reaches the end of the line, switch directions and repeat.

BALL PASS TO SIDE

Instructions

- Standing in a circle, pass the ball with both hands to the person on the right. That person should grab the ball with both hands as well. Once the ball is passed around the circle, switch directions.

GROUP BALANCE EXERCISES
SITTING IN A CIRCLE

Be sure that participants are sitting close enough to one another to perform the exercises safely.

PASS THE TRAY

Instructions

- Pass an empty tray to the next person. Gradually add objects and weight to the tray and continue passing it to the next person. Reverse directions.

OBJECT PICK-UP

Instructions

- Place six small objects such as plastic ice cubes, dice, or pens in front of each participant. Call out various numbers or colors of the objects to be picked up. After all objects are off the floor, have the participants place the objects back in front of them. Repeat the series three to five times.

SIDE PICK-UP

Instructions

- Place a can (or bottle) to the right of each participant. Instruct the participants to lean over to the right and pick up the can. Place the can in the left hand and slowly lean over to the left and set the can down on the floor. Repeat by picking up the can on the right and placing it down on the left. Repeat until the participant's original can has returned back to him.

SITTING FOOT EXERCISES

Exercising ankles and feet improves range of motion, which will decrease falls and increase circulation in older adults. Encourage participants to perform the foot exercises throughout the day.

CIRCLE AND POINT

Instructions

- Extend right foot out and circle the ankle outward 10 times. Repeat, circling the ankle inward 10 times. Point the toes up toward the ceiling and down toward the floor 5 times. Repeat circles and points with the left foot 5 times.

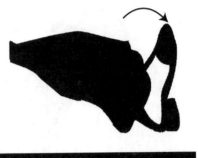

TOE AND HEEL TAP

Instructions

- Tap the soles of the right and left feet on the ground. Next, tap both heels to the ground. Repeat taps 10 times. For variety, tap the sole of the right foot and the heel of the left foot at the same time. Switch feet, tapping the right heel and the left sole. Repeat 10 times.

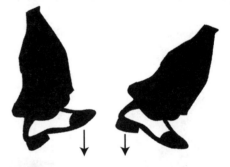

FOOT ROLL

Instructions

- Place the sole of the right foot on top of a ball or dumbbell. Slowly roll the foot forward and backward 10 times. Repeat, rolling with the left foot.

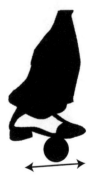

SCRUNCH AND WIGGLE

Instructions

- Scrunch the toes of the right foot toward the sole of the foot. Relax. Repeat 10 times. Scrunch the toes of the left foot toward the sole of the foot. Relax. Repeat 10 times. Scrunch the toes on both feet 10 times. Wiggle toes on the right foot 10 times. Repeat, wiggling the toes on the left foot 10 times.

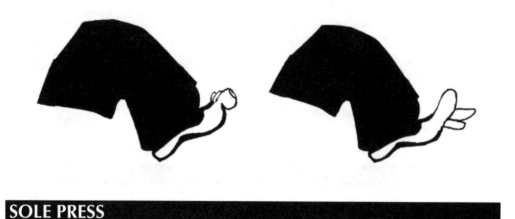

SOLE PRESS

Instructions

- Press the sole of the right foot into the floor. Hold for three seconds. Relax. Repeat, pressing 10 times.
- Press the sole of the left foot into the floor. Hold for three seconds. Relax. Repeat, pressing 10 times.

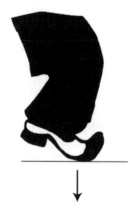

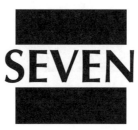

SEVEN

Program Guides

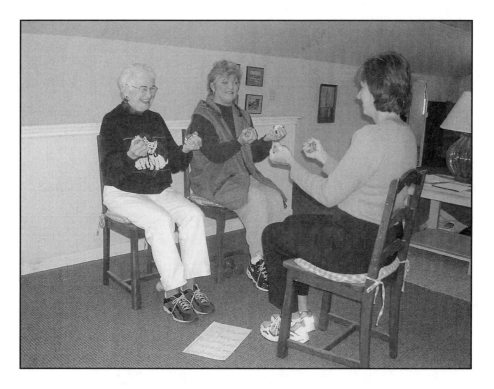

Because you may offer a variety of activity classes throughout the day, it may be difficult to recall all of the exercises to perform, not to mention the order of them. Consulting a book during class may be awkward. This chapter provides a summary for each of the Functional Fitness exercise programs. You can make a copy of each exercise program that you want to use, and you can place it in front of you to use as a visual guide.

The following are instructions for making a program guide for the exercise programs you will be using:

1.   Make a copy of both pages of the exercise program on plain copier paper.

2.   Enlarge each side to 11 by 17 inches, making these enlarged copies on colorful paper. Use a different color of paper for each program.

3.   Place both pages of each program together (using the colored copies, of course), back-to-back, and then laminate each pair together to make one exercise placemat for each program.

The staff at a local print shop or office supply store can help you to produce the program guides. Familiarize yourself thoroughly with the details of the programs in chapters 4 to 6 before you attempt to lead them.

Lift to Function Exercise Program

Warm-Up

Shoulder circles
Neck stretch

Arm stretch
Back squeeze

Wrist circles and extensions
Ball squeeze

Sitting Exercises

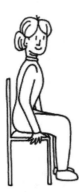

Arm press and pull

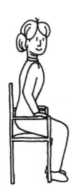

Chair lift

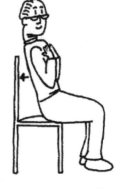

Reverse curl

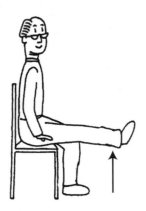

Leg extension

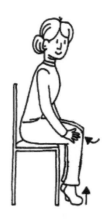

Leg squeeze

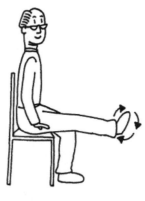

Circle and point

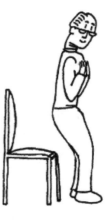

Chair stand

From *Functional Fitness for Older Adults* by Patricia A. Brill, 2004, Champaign, IL: Human Kinetics.

Lower-Body Exercises

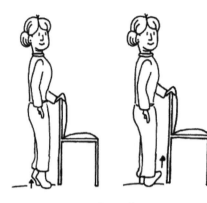 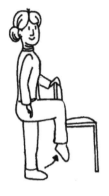 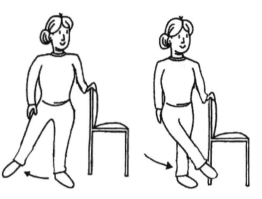

Heel and toe　　　　**Knee raise**　　　　**Leg to side and cross**

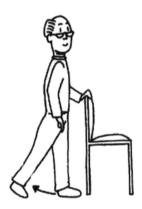 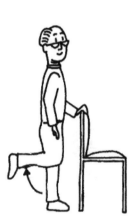 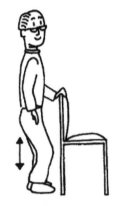

Leg to back　　　　**Leg curl**　　　　**Squats**

Cool-Down

Shoulder circles　　　Back squeeze　　　Wrist circles and extensions
Arm push　　　　　　Hugs　　　　　　Deep breathing

From *Functional Fitness for Older Adults* by Patricia A. Brill, 2004, Champaign, IL: Human Kinetics.　**109**

Squeeze to Function Exercise Program

Warm-Up

Shoulder circles Arm stretch Wrist circles
Neck stretch Arm push Chair stand

Upper-Body Exercises

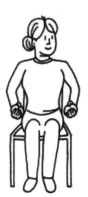

Ball squeeze

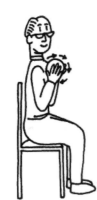

Roll and press

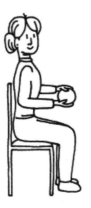

Top and bottom

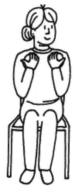

Shoulder squeeze

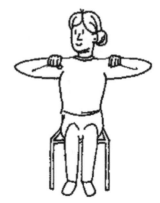

Lateral raise

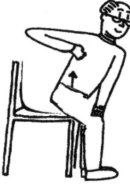

One-arm row

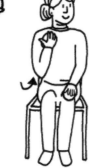

Biceps curl

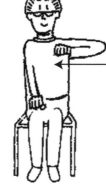
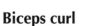

Wiper

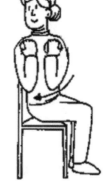

Reverse curl

Abdominal twist

Lower-Body Exercises

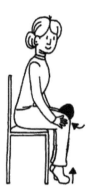
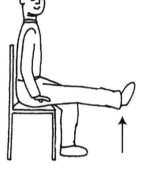
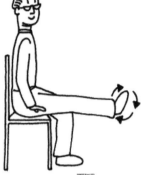
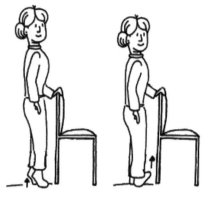

Leg squeeze   **Leg extension**   **Circle and point**   **Heel and toe**

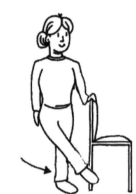
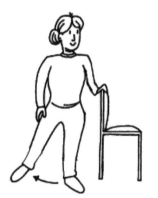
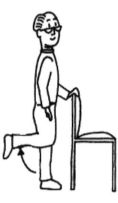

Leg to side and cross   **Leg curl**   **Squats**

Cool-Down

Shoulder circles   Back squeeze   Wrist circles and extensions
Arm push   Hugs   Deep breathing

Strengthen to Function Exercise Program

Warm-Up

Shoulder circles   Arm stretch   Wrist circles and extensions
Neck stretch   Back squeeze   Ball squeeze

Upper-Body Exercises

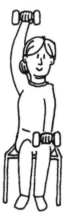

Shoulder press

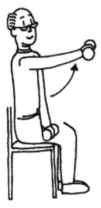

Front raise

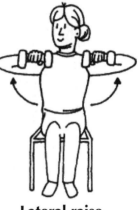

Lateral raise

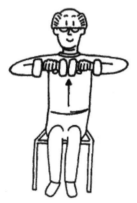

Upright row

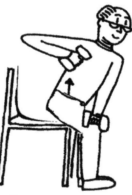

One-arm row

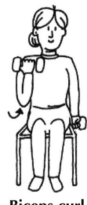

Biceps curl

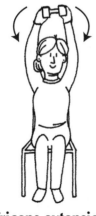

Triceps extension

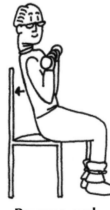

Reverse curl

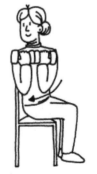

Abdominal twist

Lower-Body Exercises

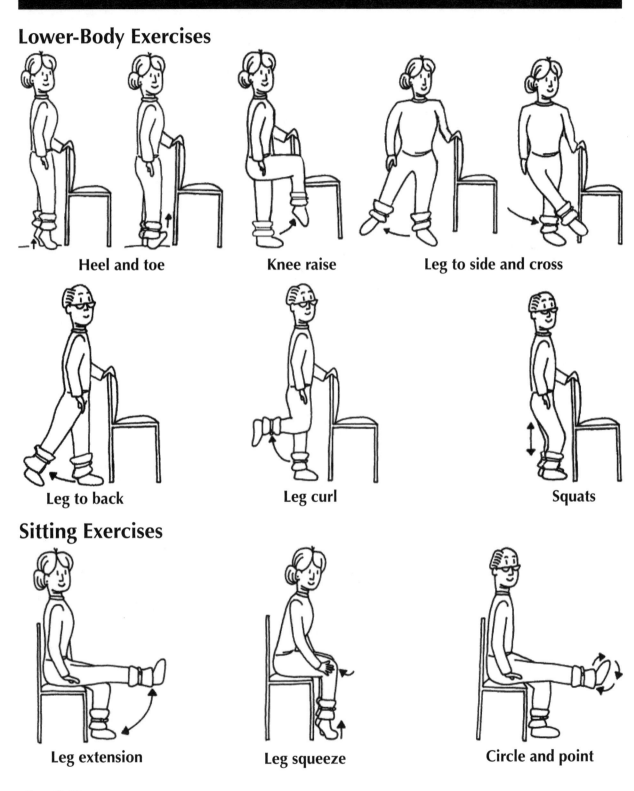

Heel and toe   **Knee raise**   **Leg to side and cross**

Leg to back   **Leg curl**   **Squats**

Sitting Exercises

Leg extension   **Leg squeeze**   **Circle and point**

Cool-Down

Shoulder circles   Back squeeze   Wrist circles and extensions
Arm push   Hugs   Deep breathing

Balance to Function Exercise Program

Warm-Up

Shoulder circles	Arm stretch	Back squeeze
Neck stretch	Arm push	Wrist circles and extensions

Individual Balance Exercises

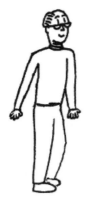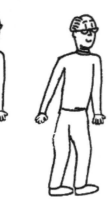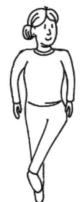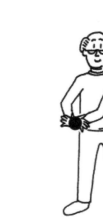

3-Stance   **Foot stand**

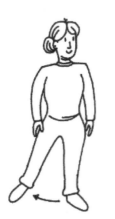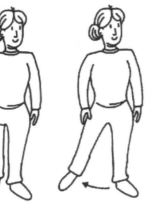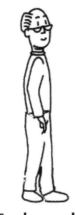

Step right and left   **Ball pass**

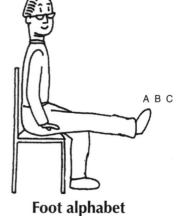

Tandem walk   **Foot alphabet**

Group Exercises Standing in a Line

Overhead ball pass   Alternate head and legs
Ball pass between legs   Ball pass to side

Group Exercises Sitting in a Circle

Pass the tray   Side pick-up
Object pick-up

Cool-Down

Shoulder circles   Back squeeze   Wrist circles and extensions
Arm push   Hugs   Deep breathing

Warm-Up and Cool-Down Exercises

Perform three to five repetitions of each exercise before and after each walk.

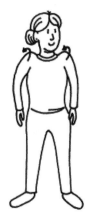 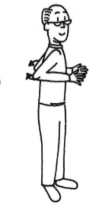 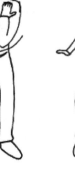 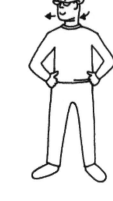 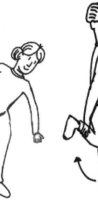 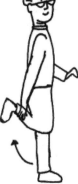

Shoulder circles   **Neck stretch**   **Back squeeze**   **Abdominal twist**   **Side bends**   **Quadriceps stretch**

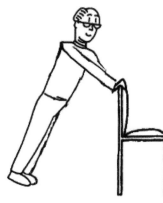 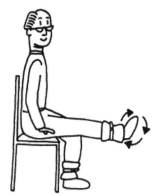 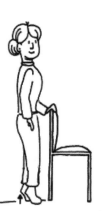 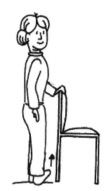

Calf stretch   **Circle and point**   **Heel and toe**

From *Functional Fitness for Older Adults* by Patricia A. Brill, 2004, Champaign, IL: Human Kinetics.

Guidelines

Stand up straight with the chin up while walking.
Swing arms at a 90-degree angle.
Maintain a good stride while walking.
Breathe evenly while walking.
Add time and distance to goals.
Try to walk 20 to 30 minutes a day.

Safety Tips

Wear comfortable, supportive walking shoes.
Walk on even, hard surfaces.
Do not walk alone, especially at night.
Do not walk during extreme heat, humidity, or cold.
Warm up and cool down before and after each walk.
Drink plenty of water before, during, and after each walk.

Step Up to Function Exercise Program

Warm-Up

Shoulder circles	Arm stretch	Back squeeze
Neck stretch	Arm push	Wrist circles and extensions

Foot Exercises

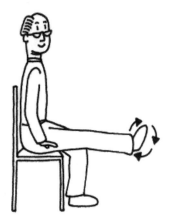

Circle and point

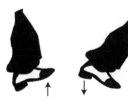

Toe and heel tap

Foot roll

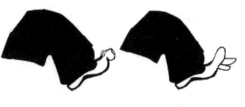

Scrunch and wiggle

Sole press

Step-Up Routine 1

Perform the appropriate step-up routine from the 12-Week Stepping Program, step-up routine 1 (page 60), starting with the right foot.

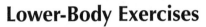

Lower-Body Exercises

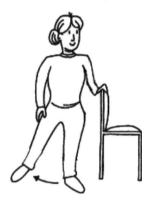
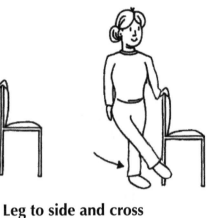
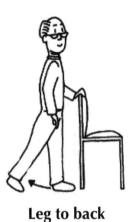
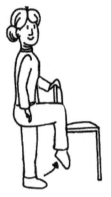

Leg to side and cross   **Leg to back**   **Knee raise**

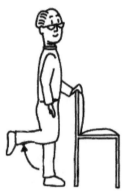
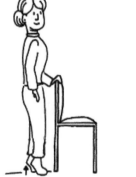
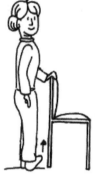
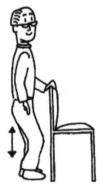

Leg curl   **Heel and toe**   **Squats**

Step-Up Routine 2

Perform the appropriate step-up routine from the 12-Week Stepping Program, step-up routine 2 (page 60), starting with the left foot.

Cool-Down

Shoulder circles   Back squeeze   Wrist circles and extensions
Arm push   Hugs   Deep breathing

Hold It to Function Exercise Program

Before beginning exercises, talk about successes or problems and provide guidelines and support.

Pelvic Floor Exercises

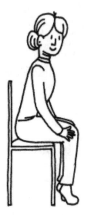

Three sets of 5 to 10 Kegels

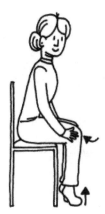

Leg squeeze

Sitting Exercises

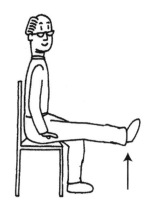

Leg extension

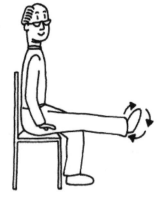

Circle and point

From *Functional Fitness for Older Adults* by Patricia A. Brill, 2004, Champaign, IL: Human Kinetics.

Standing Exercises

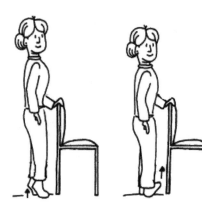
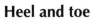

Heel and toe

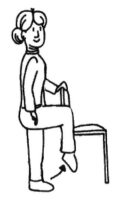

Knee raise

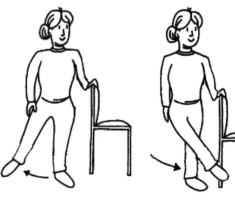

Leg to side and cross

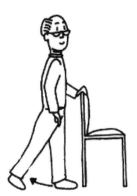

Leg to back

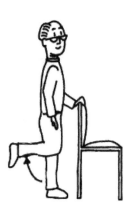

Leg curl

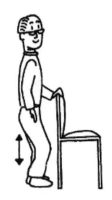

Squats

Kegels

Two sets of 5 to 10 Kegels

Move to Function Exercise Program

Upper-Body Exercises

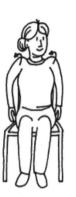 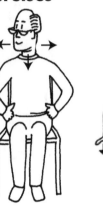 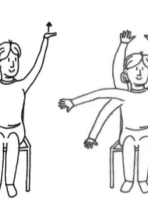 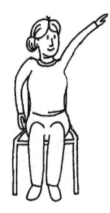

Shoulder circles **Neck stretch** **Arm stretch** **Arm push** **Arm circles**

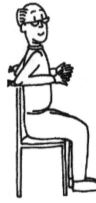 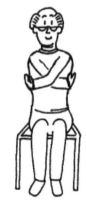 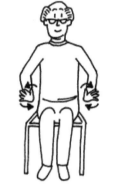 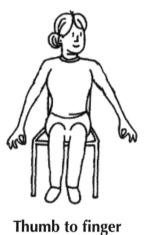

Back squeeze **Hugs** **Wrist circles and extensions** **Thumb to finger**

Lower-Body Exercises

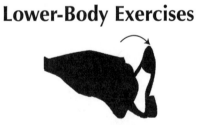 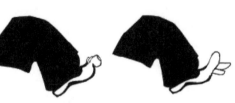

Circle and point **Scrunch and wiggle**

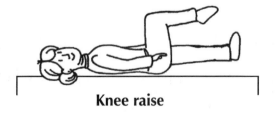 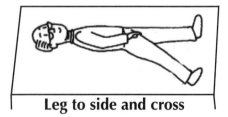

Knee raise **Leg to side and cross**

Ball Exercises

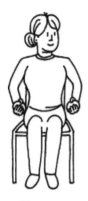

Ball squeeze

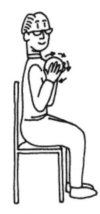

Roll and press

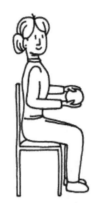

Top and bottom press

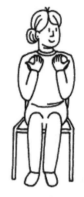

Shoulder squeeze

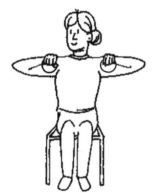

Lateral raise

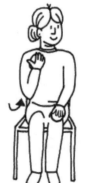

One-arm row

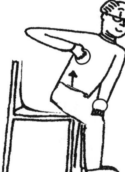

Biceps curl

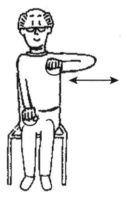

Wiper

Remember to Function Exercise Program

Warm-Up

Shoulder circles	Arm stretch	Wrist circles	Circle and point
Neck stretch	Hugs	Leg extension	Heel and toe

Large Ball Exercises

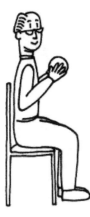 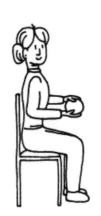 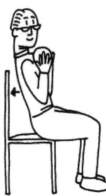 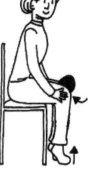 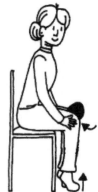

Side press   **Top and bottom press**   **Reverse curl**   **Leg squeeze**

Small Ball Exercises

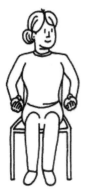 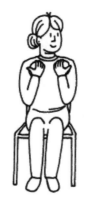 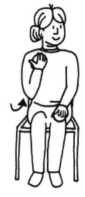

Ball squeeze   **Roll and press**   **Shoulder squeeze**   **Biceps curl**

Pick up all of the balls and clear the area.

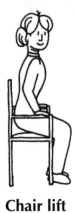

Chair lift

It's time to stand up and perform the leg exercises. Participants with poor balance should sit and exercise. Participants standing should hold onto the back of a chair.

Standing Exercises

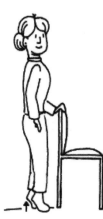

Heel and toe

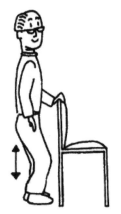

Leg to side

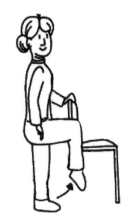

Squats

Marching

Cool-Down

Shoulder circles
Arm stretch

Arm push
Hugs

Wrist circles and extensions
Deep breathing

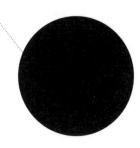

HOLD IT TO FUNCTION

Perform the following exercises daily.

Stop and Hold
While you are urinating, stop the flow and hold for 2 seconds. Release the flow, then stop and hold again.

Kegel Exercises
Perform 20 to 30 Kegel exercises two to three times daily. You can perform these exercises while watching TV, driving, or reading.

How to perform Kegel exercises:
Squeeze in the rectum. Next, squeeze up as strongly as possible the entire pelvic floor, as if you are trying to stop the flow of urine. Hold for 3 seconds. Relax, then repeat.

Decrease Your Risk for Incontinence
- Limit consumption of caffeine and alcoholic drinks.
- Consume 6 to 8 glasses of water daily.
- Consume a diet high in fiber, fruits, and vegetables.
- Exercise on a regular basis.
- Perform Kegel exercises daily.
- Don't smoke. (Nicotine can irritate the bladder.)
- Urinate on a regular basis.

From *Functional Fitness for Older Adults* by Patricia A. Brill, 2004, Champaign, IL: Human Kinetics.

HOLD IT TO FUNCTION

Perform 10 repetitions of each exercise one to two times per day.

Strengthening lower-body muscles will improve mobility and balance, thus allowing you to get to the bathroom in time once an urge hits.

Squats

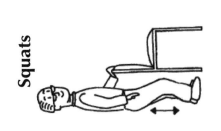

Leg to back

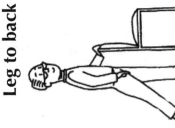
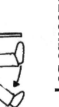
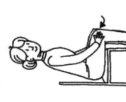

Leg to side and cross

Leg squeeze

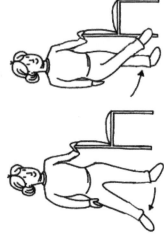

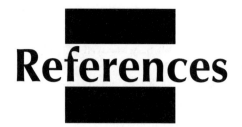

References

ACSM Position Stand on Exercise and Physical Activity for Older Adults. 1998. *Medicine and Science in Sports and Exercise, 30* (6): 992-1008.

American Senior Fitness Association. (1994). *Long term care fitness leader training manual* (1st ed.). New Smyrna Beach, FL: American Senior Fitness Association.

American Senior Fitness Association. (2003). *Senior fitness instructor training manual* (6th ed.). New Smyrna Beach, FL: American Senior Fitness Association.

American Senior Fitness Association. (2004). *Special population imperatives for custom older adult training* (4th ed.). New Smyrna Beach, FL: American Senior Fitness Association.

Brill, P.A., Drimmer, A.M., Morgan, L.A., & Gordon, N.F. (1995). Feasibility of conducting strength and flexibility programs in elderly nursing home residents with dementia. *The Gerontologist, 35:* 263-266.

Brill, P.A., Jensen, R.L., Koltyn, K.F., Morgan, L.A., Morrow, J.R., Keller, M.J., & Jackson, A.W. (1998). The feasibility of conducting a group-based strength training program in residents of a multi-level care facility. *Activities, Adaptation, and Aging, 22* (4): 53-63.

Brill, P.A., Macera, C.A., Davis, D.R., Blair, S.N., & Gordon, N.F. (2000). Muscular strength and physical function. *Medicine and Science in Sports and Exercise, 32* (2): 412-416.

Brill, P.A., Matthews, M., Mason, J., Davis, D., Mustafa, T., & Macera, C.A. (1998). Improving functional performance through a group-based free weight strength training program in residents of assisted living programs. *Physical and Occupational Therapy in Geriatrics, 15* (3): 57-69.

Brill, P.A., Probst, J.C., Greenhouse, D.L., Schell, B., & Macera, C.A. (1998). Improving functional capability through a cost-effective functional fitness strength training program. *The Journal of the American Board of Family Practice, 11* (6): 445-451.

Brill, P.A. (1999). Effective approach toward prevention and rehabilitation in geriatrics. *Activities, Adaptation, and Aging, 23* (4): 21-32.

Decker, J., & Mize, M. (2002). *Walking games and activities: 40 new ways to make fitness fun.* Champaign, IL: Human Kinetics.

Fiatarone, M.A., Marks, E.C., Ryan, N.D., Meredith, C.N., Lipsitz, L.A., & Evans, W.J. (1990). High-intensity strength training in nonagenarians. *Journal of the American Medical Association, 263:* 3029-3034.

Fiatarone, M.A., O'Neill, E.F., Ryan, N.D., Clements, K.M., Solares, G.R., Nelson, M.E., Roberts, S.B., Kehayias, J.J., Lipsitz, L.A., & Evans, W.J. (1994). Exercise training and nutritional supplementation for physical frailty in very elderly people. *New England Journal of Medicine, 330:* 1769-1775.

Fisher, N.M., Pendergast, D.R., & Calkins, E. (1991). Muscle rehabilitation in impaired elderly nursing home residents. *Archives of Physical Medicine and Rehabilitation, 72:* 181-185.

Frontera, W.R., Meredith, C.N., O'Reilly, K.P., Knuttgen, H.G., & Evans, W.J. (1988). Strength conditioning in older men: Skeletal muscle hypertrophy and improved function. *Journal of Applied Physiology, 64:* 1038-1044.

Gillespie, L.D., Gillespie, W.J., Robertson, M.C., et al. (2002). Interventions for preventing falls in elderly people (Cochrane Review). In: *The Cochrane Library*, Issue 2. Oxford: Update Software.

Huang, Y., Macera, C.A., Blair, S.N., Brill, P.A., Kohl, H.W., & Kroenfeld, J.J. (1998). Physical fitness, physical activity and functional limitations in older adults. *Medicine and Science in Sports and Exercise, 30* (9): 1430-1435.

Hyatt, R.H., Ehitelow, M.N., Bhat, A., Scott, S., & Maxwell, J.D. (1990). Association of muscle strength with functional status of elderly people. *Age and Ageing, 19:* 330-336.

King, A.C., Pruitt, L.A., Phillips, W., Oka, R., Rodenburg, A., & Haskell, W.L. (2000). Comparative effects of two physical activity programs on measured and perceived physical functioning and other health-related quality of life outcomes in older adults. *Journals of Gerontology: Series A, Biological Sciences and Medical Sciences, 55* (2): M74-83.

Petrella, R.J. (1999). Exercises for older patients with chronic disease. *The Physician and Sportsmedicine, 7* (11). Champaign, IL: Human Kinetics.

Rikli, R., & Jones, C. (2001). *Senior fitness test manual.* Champaign, IL: Human Kinetics.

Rikli, R., & Jones, C. (2001). *Senior fitness test video.* Champaign, IL: Human Kinetics.

Thompson, R.F., Crist, D.M., Marsh, M., & Rosenthal, M. (1988). Effects of physical exercise for elderly patients with physical impairments. *Journal of the American Geriatrics Society, 36:* 130-135.

US Department of Health and Human Services (1996). *Physical activity and health: A report of the Surgeon General.* Atlanta, Georgia: US Department of Health and Human Services, Public Health Service, CDC, National Center for Chronic Disease Prevention and Health Promotion.

Williams, R.D. (1997). Medications and older adults. *US Food and Drug Administration Consumer Magazine, 5.*

Wood, R.H., Reyes, R., Welsch, M.A., Favaloro-Sabatier, J., Sabatier, M., Matthew, L.C., Johnson, L.G., & Hooper, P.F. (2001). Concurrent cardiovascular and resistance training in healthy older adults. *Medicine and Science in Sports Exercise, 33* (10): 1751-1758.

About the Author

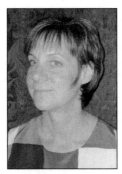

Patricia A. Brill, PhD, is the founder of Functional Fitness, L.L.C., a consulting company that designs and implements fitness and wellness programs for seniors. She has developed and produced 4 exercise and training videos for seniors as well as 10 functional fitness exercise programs with accompanying illustrated guides. For the last decade, she has conducted research and designed exercise programs for older adults living at home, in independent and assisted living communities, or in nursing homes, as well as in dementia care facilities. Older adults' regular participation in these exercise programs has resulted in their being able to walk, travel, bathe, dress themselves, and perform many social and physical activities they were previously unable to participate in.

In 1998, Dr. Brill was awarded the American College of Sports Medicine Healthy People 2000 Physical Activity Promotion Award for designing and implementing a research strength training program for a large assisted-living corporation. In 1997, she was awarded the South Carolina Governor's Award for Research in Aging for the design and implementation of a placemat that illustrates a strength-training program called "The Kitchen Table Is Not Just for Eating . . . Let's Exercise." Dr. Brill also was presented with the University of South Carolina's Award for Excellence in Research for the 1994-1995 academic year for the creation of a Functional Fitness Strength Training Program to Restore Activities of Daily Living in Frail Individuals. In 2001 she won the National Mature Media Award for her training video on dementia and exercise.

Dr. Brill is a fellow of the American College of Sports Medicine. She has published more than 25 peer-reviewed research articles, coauthored a fitness prescription provider guide for physicians and health professionals, and has presented on exercise for older adults at more than 15 national conferences.

In her free time, Dr. Brill enjoys boating, traveling, and listening to blues music. She resides in Houston, Texas.

Dr. Brill's exercise and training videos that accompany some of the Functional Fitness for Older Adults exercise programs can be ordered from Functional Fitness, L.L.C at www.muscles2function.com.